THE ESSENTIALS OF
NURSING
LEADERSHIP

SAGE was founded in 1965 by Sara Miller McCune to support the dissemination of usable knowledge by publishing innovative and high-quality research and teaching content. Today, we publish over 900 journals, including those of more than 400 learned societies, more than 800 new books per year, and a growing range of library products including archives, data, case studies, reports, and video. SAGE remains majority-owned by our founder, and after Sara's lifetime will become owned by a charitable trust that secures our continued independence.

Los Angeles | London | New Delhi | Singapore | Washington DC | Melbourne

THE ESSENTIALS OF
NURSING LEADERSHIP

RUTH TAYLOR & BRIAN WEBSTER-HENDERSON

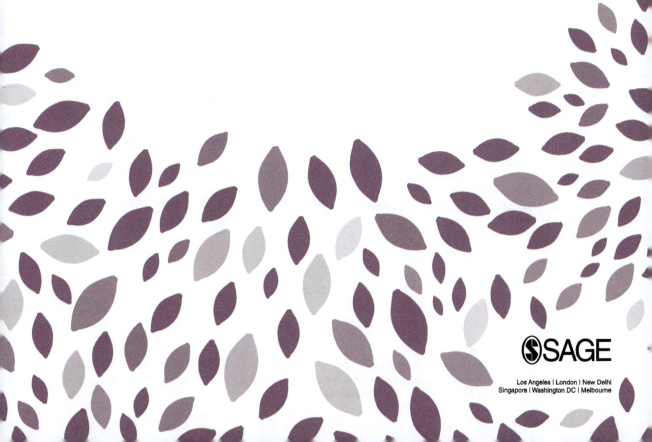

$SAGE

Los Angeles | London | New Delhi
Singapore | Washington DC | Melbourne

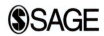

Los Angeles | London | New Delhi
Singapore | Washington DC | Melbourne

SAGE Publications Ltd
1 Oliver's Yard
55 City Road
London EC1Y 1SP

SAGE Publications Inc.
2455 Teller Road
Thousand Oaks, California 91320

SAGE Publications India Pvt Ltd
B 1/I 1 Mohan Cooperative Industrial Area
Mathura Road
New Delhi 110 044

SAGE Publications Asia-Pacific Pte Ltd
3 Church Street
#10-04 Samsung Hub
Singapore 049483

Editor: Becky Taylor
Editorial assistant: Charlène Burin
Production editor: Katie Forsythe
Copyeditor: Andy Baxter
Proofreader: Audrey Scriven
Indexer: Elske Janssen
Marketing manager: Tamara Navaratnam
Cover design: Wendy Scott
Typeset by: C&M Digitals (P) Ltd, Chennai, India
Printed in the UK

First edition published 2017

Library of Congress Control Number: 2016940070

British Library Cataloguing in Publication data

A catalogue record for this book is available from the British
Library

ISBN 978-1-4129-6201-8
ISBN 978-1-4129-6202-5 (pbk)

At SAGE we take sustainability seriously. Most of our products are printed in the UK using FSC papers and boards.
When we print overseas we ensure sustainable papers are used as measured by the PREPS grading system.
We undertake an annual audit to monitor our sustainability.

This book is dedicated to all the student nurses and registered nurses who aspire to provide the highest quality of nursing care and who make a positive difference to the patients and clients they meet every day and throughout their careers.

CONTENTS

ABOUT THE
EDITORS AND
CONTRIBUTORS

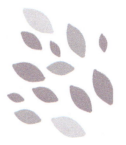

Ruth Taylor is Professor of Nursing and Pro Vice Chancellor and Dean of the Faculty of Health, Social Care and Education at Anglia Ruskin University. Ruth is a nurse by background and worked as an oncology nurse and general practice nurse in the UK and New Zealand. She moved into higher education around 18 years ago and has worked in a variety of roles including course leadership, Deputy Dean and now as Dean. Ruth was awarded a professorship in 2012, in part for her work on the student experience and her leadership and impact at a national level. She is a Florence Nightingale Foundation Leadership scholar and is passionate about the development of leadership in others. Ruth is a member of a number of national and international bodies, including as a member of the Executive Team for the UK Council of Deans of Health. She has connections that span professions, geography and expertise. Ruth has published across a range of areas including networking, leadership, the student experience and compassion in healthcare.

Brian Webster-Henderson is University Dean of Learning and Teaching and Professor of Nursing at Edinburgh Napier University. Prior to this, Brian worked in a number of senior roles in nursing and midwifery in the UK including Head of the School of Nursing and Midwifery at Robert Gordon University, Aberdeen, and as Director of Education at the School of Nursing and Midwifery, University of Southampton. He is both a mental health nurse and an adult nurse and has been in nursing since leaving school. His clinical career has spread across a number of areas including alcohol services, elderly care, cancer care and medical nursing. He worked as a lecturer–practitioner before moving into higher education full time in 1997. Brian speaks regularly on issues pivotal to nurse education both in the UK and overseas, and is Vice Chair of the Council of Deans of Health UK as well as Convenor of the Council of Deans of Health (Scotland).

Tim Bryson is an independent healthcare consultant, having formerly worked for ten years as Executive Director of Nursing for Cambridgeshire and Peterborough NHS Foundation Trust. From 2012 to 2015 Tim worked for Cambridge University Health Partners on education developments, including leadership programme development.

Tim has a strong interest in leadership development and his MSc dissertation focused on a leadership analysis of the National Service Framework for Mental Health. Tim is currently project manager for a regional health foundation project on patient safety, and heading up a service for adolescents with Essex County Council.

Sandra Cairncross is an Assistant Principal at Edinburgh Napier University, with a specific focus on the student experience. Within this role she has led the development of the Edinburgh Napier Student Experience Strategy which has an emphasis on providing opportunities for students to apply learning and develop transferable skills outside the classroom. Sandra favours a coaching approach to leadership and is committed to her ongoing development as a leader. She is also a member of the Leadership Foundation in Higher Education's Membership Advisory Board. She completed her PhD 'Interactive Multimedia: Realising the Benefits' part time and remains active in pedagogical research. Current interests focus on exploring student engagement outside the classroom with an emphasis on promoting equality and diversity.

Alison Crombie was, until recently, the Executive Director of Education and Quality for Health Education Kent, Surrey and Sussex Local Education and Training Board. Previously she was a director of education in a large acute trust in London bringing together education services across hospitals and sites under one multi-professional directorate. Her post was a joint academic professorial role supporting research and educational activity across professions. Much of Alison's focus has been on working in and with challenged trusts to use education and research strategies to develop solutions to promote team working, changes in workforce and innovation in the delivery of safer care across care pathways. Alison is a qualified coach, academic supervisor and mentor for the national leadership programme.

Jayne Donaldson is the Dean of the Faculty of Health Sciences and Sport at the University of Stirling, and Professor of Nursing. She is a nurse by background, a member of the Council of Deans of Health Scotland, and has a keen interest in the quality of patient experience within healthcare, and the development of leadership knowledge and skills in the healthcare workforce. For example, she has developed work for NHS Education for Scotland, including *Flying Start*, an online web-based programme for all newly qualified nurses, midwives and allied health professionals in Scotland, and chaired a group which developed an online learning resource, *Compassionate Connections*, which aims to improve compassionate care within healthcare provision in maternity services across Scotland.

Gayle Garland is a Senior Lecturer at the School of Healthcare at the University of Leeds and programme leader for the Master of Leadership and Management in Health and Social Care. She has a special interest in frontline leadership and its impact on patient care and experience. She led on the national frontline leadership programme *Leadership at the Point of Care* and was a vital part of the team that delivered the national *Leading* *an Empowered Organisation* programme in England. Gayle's professional nursing career originated in Canada and expanded to include clinical and management experiences in California before she came to the UK. She brings experiences of diverse healthcare systems and approaches and has a talent for translating complex issues into practice.

Mary Gobbi is a Professorial Fellow in Nursing Education, in the Faculty of Health Sciences at the University of Southampton. Her research and educational interests relate to the development of healthcare expertise and competence, and professional capital with a particular focus in simulation and tacit knowledge. She leads a doctoral module on service improvement and innovation. Her clinical background is in critical care nursing, specifically cardio-thoracic and vascular. Mary is a member of several international groups including the Tuning Academy. She is an international commissioner for the American Nurses Association and undertakes a range of advisory roles/ projects at national and international levels.

Lizzie Jelfs is Director of the Council of Deans of Health, the representative voice of the UK's university faculties engaged in education and research for nursing, midwifery and the allied health professions. She has worked in health policy roles for the past eight years but began her career on the NHS Management Training Scheme and worked in the NHS before moving to Brussels, where she was Deputy Director of the European Health Management Association. Lizzie read modern history at Oxford University and holds an MSc in health leadership and management from Birmingham and Manchester Universities.

Gillian McCready qualified as an executive coach in 2003, following a career in leadership and organisation development within the financial services and manufacturing sectors. She has coached over 300 managers, directors and CEOs as an independent consultant and qualified as a supervisor in 2009. Gillian has recently completed a year's programme, 'Developing Excellence in Supervision', with the Gestalt Psychotherapy Institute to deepen her practice. She provides team coaching to leadership teams, and designs and facilitates workshops to develop coaching as a management style. She is an accredited 'Time to Think' facilitator. Gillian has an honours degree in psychology and postgraduate qualifications in teaching, education and personnel management.

Mike Sabin is an experienced nurse and educator who has worked in education, policy development and clinical practice in NHS Scotland. From his clinical background in critical care, Mike moved into nursing education and then into senior roles in educational quality assurance, commissioning and health policy. His particular areas of interest span student recruitment and retention, clinical leadership, advanced practice and supporting numeracy skills in healthcare practice.

Stephen Tee joined Bournemouth University as Executive Dean of the Faculty of Health and Social Sciences in September 2015. He is a Professor of Nurse Education.

Stephen has held senior leadership roles in higher education in organisations such as King's College and the University of Southampton. He has worked in the NHS and in higher education for 30 years and has provided strategic and operational leadership in a range of senior roles. His research interests include participatory approaches to healthcare delivery and education, particularly focusing on service user involvement. He has published widely on many aspects of nurse education in healthcare and has edited books and journals. He was appointed Principal Fellow of King's College London and the Higher Education Academy in 2014 and was made a National Teaching Fellow in 2015.

Annette Thomas-Gregory is currently Head of the Department of Nursing and Midwifery, Cambridge at Anglia Ruskin University. She is a nurse by background and specialised in haematology, oncology and palliative care nursing, making the move into higher education when an opportunity arose to develop cancer and palliative care education within Cambridgeshire. Since working in higher education, Annette has completed a Master's degree at London Southbank University, and an educational doctorate at Leicester University. Annette believes that these exceptional educational experiences have furnished her with role-specific skills, and developed her confidence and ability to think critically and to demonstrate evidence-informed ethical leadership.

Susan Tokley has been a registered nurse for over 35 years and a registered health visitor for more than 20 years. She is also an experienced coach, Myers Briggs practitioner, a mentor and a Florence Nightingale Leadership Scholar. She has held a number of senior and strategic director level nursing roles in acute, community and commissioning and policy organisations during the last 20 years at national, regional and local levels. She is currently an independent nurse consultant. Her main interests and expertise are in health service management, professional and organisational development, and clinical leadership. She is currently Vice Chair of the Executive Nurse Network in London.

FOREWORD

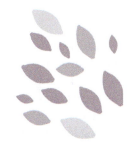

I am delighted to write the Foreword for this important textbook on the essentials of leadership for student nurses. As Chief Executive of the Florence Nightingale Foundation and of course as a nurse and midwife, I am passionate about the need for leaders who behave with integrity, intelligence, compassion and courage. However long you have been a student nurse, I am sure that you will have seen the changes and the challenges that affect healthcare delivery. One of our biggest healthcare challenges is to develop the leadership capacity and capability of the workforce with nurses front and centre of that leadership challenge. How do we make this a reality? In part it is through the experience and knowledge of our current leaders; but it is also through our future and aspiring leaders who will make a sustainable difference to the future of nursing practice. This is where you as a student nurse come in. I share the authors' view that student nurses are developing leaders in their own right as soon as they step into clinical practice. To the public and those that you are entrusted to care for, you are seen immediately as a person with knowledge and the ability to provide help, support and give professional care to those individuals at their most vulnerable time. The smallest interactions can have the biggest impact, and what you do every day when you are in practice will make the difference to many individuals one person at a time.

You will, no doubt, be as committed as I am to seeing nursing and midwifery practice that leads to better outcomes and an improving experience for patients. It is this commitment that can lead you to realise your potential as a student and into qualified practice. This textbook offers you a theoretical overview – taking you through the relevant knowledge that you will need as you develop as a leader. The book does two other things: it offers you practical tools and skills that you can develop across a range of important leadership behaviours (coaching, networking, and reflection amongst others). Uniquely, it also speaks to you using the voices of nurse leaders and student nurses who offer insights into their own leadership journeys and what they see as important for professional leadership. I think you will find these extremely useful as you think about the theory and its application to your own practice.

I am proud to see the impact of the work of the Florence Nightingale Foundation through this book. The Foundation exists to support nurses through scholarships and mentorship as well as recognition for the work that they do every day in making positive differences to people's lives. Ruth Taylor (one of the editors) and two of the nursing/midwifery leaders (Tracy Humphrey and Debbie Carreck-Sen) are previous or current Florence Nightingale Foundation scholars. Their scholarships have enabled them to work towards the achievement of their leadership potential and to make a difference in practice through their work as educators, researchers, and practitioners. As the Chief Executive of the Foundation, I am privileged to see first-hand the difference that leaders make to individuals and organisations through our leadership scholarships.

I do hope that you will enjoy using this book. Pick it up when you need some inspiration from student nurses who, like you, are developing as leaders. Dip into it when you come across challenging situations in practice and need to reflect on how leadership can make a positive difference to healthcare. Finally, try and encompass the values of 'good' leadership and make a difference every day.

Professor Elizabeth Robb OBE
Chief Executive
The Florence Nightingale Foundation

ACKNOWLEDGEMENTS

Ruth and Brian would like to thank all those individuals who have contributed to this book. Your involvement and influence will be appreciated by many readers – thank you.

PUBLISHER'S ACKNOWLEDGEMENTS

The publishers would like to thank the following individuals for their invaluable feedback on the proposal and draft chapters:

Melody Carter, La Trobe University, Australia

Mary Casey, University College Dublin, Ireland

Stephanie Dunleavy, Ulster University, Ireland

Judith Enterkin, London Southbank University, UK

Caia Francis, University of the West of England, UK

Irene Kennedy, Glasgow Caledonian University, UK

Claire Smith, Sheffield Teaching Hospitals NHS Foundation Trust, UK

We would also like to thank the nurse leaders, as well as the students below who were involved in the book – it is much richer for your contribution.

Clare Benney

Laura Berrill

Briannie Falconer

Hannah Leggett

Louisa McGee

Carol Roughley

Lorraine Thompsett

Amy Tran

Emma Wolton

The authors and publishers are grateful to the following for their kind permission to reproduce material:

Table 2.1: Reproduced from 'Leadership theories and the development of nurses in primary health care', *Primary Health Care*, 19(9): 40–45 and with kind permission from *Primary Health Care*.

The author and publisher are also grateful to Burning Eye Books for their kind permission to reproduce Molly Case's poem 'Nursing the Nation', taken from her collection *Underneath the Roses Where I Remembered Everything*.

HOW TO USE THE COMPANION WEBSITE

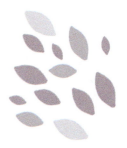

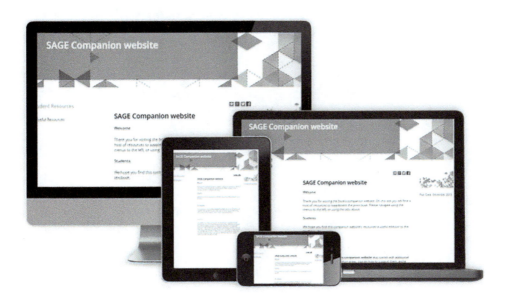

The Essentials of Nursing Leadership is supported by a wealth of online resources for both students and lecturers to aid study and support teaching, which are available at https://study.sagepub.com/taylor. Look out for the 🖱 icon throughout the book, which will remind you to access the website for the following materials.

- **Watch and learn**: Student and nurse leader video interviews show you **real-life examples** of how you can become a leader at any stage of your career.
- **Succeed at assignments**: selected **free SAGE journal articles** help you deepen your knowledge and understanding of key topics.
- **Keep ahead**: weblinks to policy documents and other relevant resources help you have **the latest information at your fingertips**.

INTRODUCTION

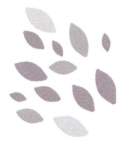

The book roadmap and core skills for leadership

Ruth Taylor and Brian Webster-Henderson

To find out more about Ruth and Brian, please visit the companion website at https:study.sagepub.com/taylor

INTRODUCTION

Welcome to our edited book on leadership in nursing. As editors, we are delighted to bring to you a new approach to talking about leadership. We believe that good leadership is a key component of providing good quality care to patients in a range of environments and settings. We are also of the view that leadership development, knowledge, and the rehearsal of leadership styles and skills are an important part of the student nurse's learning journey.

In recent years the nursing profession has been at the centre of media scrutiny and a changing public perception of nursing which has resulted in political scrutiny of the profession.

The scrutiny of nursing

In the past few years, there has been a growing focus from the media around the delivery of poor nursing care, in both the NHS and the private sector within the UK. Television documentaries, newspaper articles, and NHS inspections have regularly focused on a plethora of organisations where the nursing care provided to a range of patients (from the elderly to mental health and learning disability clients) has been of a very poor quality.

Public concerns about nursing

At the same time, the UK has seen a number of key public inquiries and investigations following allegations and complaints by patients and relatives about poor nursing care.

In 2013, Sir Robert Francis published his report of a public inquiry into the Mid Staffordshire NHS Trust following a series of ongoing complaints from relatives and several deaths of patients. A total of 293 recommendations were made following the findings from his investigation around a culture of poor care and poor leadership (Department of Health, 2013).

In 2014 the Scottish Government published its Vale of Leven Public Inquiry following a lengthy investigation into the deaths from *Clostridium difficile* of several patients in the Vale of Leven Hospital (Scottish Government, 2014). In both these key reports, the leadership by healthcare professionals, and in particular that of nurses, was heavily criticised.

A policy response

As a result of a number of policy responses to these and other reports, recommendations about nursing and the need for change with a consistent approach to effective leadership have been published. In 2010 the Prime Minister published a 'high level' report on the future of nursing and midwifery in the UK (Department of Health, 2010). From the 20 recommendations, effective leadership in nursing was a pivotal concern. Yet again a further review in 2015 (referred to as the 'Shape of Caring') places continued emphasis on the need for strong nursing leaders within the UK (Health Education England, 2015).

It is within this climate and context that we believe a contemporary book on leadership is required to support you as you learn, develop, rehearse and reflect on the knowledge and skills that you will require in order to be effective leaders in your chosen field of nursing. We both passionately believe that leadership development starts at the moment you commence your professional, graduate nurse education and can be developed theoretically and in practice. It will be no surprise then that the Nursing and Midwifery Council (NMC) identify leadership as a significant requirement and expectation of a student nurse's learning journey (NMC, 2010) and their professional registration (NMC, 2015). We both hope that this book will facilitate your learning and development, but in order to do so it is important that you understand how to get the best out of it.

Visit the companion website at https://study.sagepub.com/taylor to watch Ruth and Brian discussing the origins, key messages, and key features of the book, as well as giving you tips on how to be a good leader.

INTRODUCTION PURPOSE

The purpose of this introduction is to signpost you towards the structure and content of the book, the types of activities we have designed, and the ways in which you may wish to use the book in support of your learning in your university and practice placements. We have taken a similar approach to the one that Ruth took in her research textbook (*The Essentials of Nursing and Healthcare Research*: Taylor, 2012) which seemed to work well for students. Like the topic of research, some of you will be undertaking a curriculum in which leadership is threaded through all of your units or modules of learning. Others of you will be undertaking specific modules which focus on leadership (and probably management). This book is designed so you can dip into and out of it as you need – to link to a particular theoretical or practice learning experience, or simply to develop your knowledge-base as you progress through your course. We hope that the approach we have used will suit these differing needs. The authors of the chapters in this book are all leaders in their own right – some are academics with clinical backgrounds, others are clinicians or researchers, still others are managers across a spectrum of settings. Student nurses have also contributed to one of the book chapters – leaders in their own right – and we are really pleased they wanted to be a part of this project. We chose the authors carefully as our aim is to offer the knowledge required for your course in ways that are inspiring and effective. All of the authors are committed to working with students in their different work settings in ways that will enable student nurses to thrive and grow as leaders. We think that this approach comes through clearly in each of the chapters – in different ways, each one offers fresh perspectives on leadership in nursing with, for the purposes of this book, the student nurse at the centre.

The learning activities are designed to bring to the fore the perspectives of the authors – offering you a chance to consider different viewpoints, question practice, and to look at yourself as you develop in your role and your own leadership skills and attributes. We both know that being a 'good' leader is an evolving process and that as a student nurse you may not even see yourself as a leader. We want to challenge your thinking and encourage you to see why your early development as a leader will play a crucial part in improving practice. We have used examples of nursing practice across all the fields – adult, mental health, children and young people, and learning disability. So we hope that you will feel engaged with the focus of the book, and that you will use the examples we offer as a springboard to explore the issues in leadership further.

OVERVIEW OF THE BOOK'S AIMS AND OBJECTIVES

The overall aim of this book is to enable you, as a student, to develop the relevant knowledge and skills (and possibly attributes) that are needed for leadership in this evolving and volatile health and social care context. The authors have provided the theory that you will need to do this in ways that are clearly applied to different contexts in practice – so that you can see the relevance of the theory to real-life situations. In particular, we are pleased to be able to let you 'hear' the voices of student nurses and successful nurse leaders, both in the book and in the videos on the companion website (https://study.sagepub.com/taylor), so that you can appreciate their experiences and perspectives, and consider their relevance to your nursing journey.

This book will enable you to achieve the following overall objectives:

1. To develop your understanding of theories of leadership and management in healthcare practice.
2. To appreciate your role as a leader and student nurse and how you can impact positively on practice.
3. To apply knowledge of, and skills in, leadership to practice.
4. To value how your role as a leader can impact positively on the care of service users, carers and relatives, as well as on how you can be a role model for colleagues.

As a starting point, undertake the activity below – it aims to begin your thinking and to act as a benchmark for your development as you work your way through your course. You may want to come back to your notes in future.

Introduction activity

Reflect on the following points and make notes which you can come back to at a later date if you wish:

1. How would you define leadership?
2. What role do you think a student nurse has as a leader?
3. What is the importance of leadership for clinical practice?

You may have come up with a whole range of areas that you think might define leadership. Some of these may relate to inspiring others to achieve a vision, or to ensuring that things get done. As you consider the theoretical perspectives in the book, you will be able to draw your own conclusions about this and the other questions.

OVERVIEW OF THE BOOK'S CHAPTERS

Each of the chapters has a key focus and these are described below. What you will find though is that there is plenty of overlap across the chapters. Healthcare practice, and leadership for nursing and healthcare practice, are huge areas with many viewpoints, perspectives and a wide range of evidence to support those practices. The overlapping nature of the theoretical underpinnings for leadership is key to our overall understanding of how leadership is enacted in practice. We have provided signposts across chapters so that you can delve more deeply into the areas that are of particular interest to you. For ease, however, here is an overview of the key learning points within each of the chapters.

CHAPTER OUTLINES

Part One: Knowledge and theory

Chapter 1: The context of leadership in practice

This chapter offers a brief historical overview and background of nursing leadership, with some key examples of nursing leaders cited to help you see how leadership in nursing has evolved over the years. The chapter touches on the policy context in the UK – though this is covered in depth in Chapter 3 – and how that context is relevant to nursing leadership in our current healthcare and political context. Linked to this, the author introduces the student nurse as a leader, so that you can start to make some connections between what goes on at policy level, and what you are doing as you learn in your clinical placements. Your role as a student undertaking a degree – with the recent move to an all-graduate profession across the UK – is highlighted.

Chapter 2: Nursing leadership in organisations: Theory and practice

A book on leadership would not be complete without definitions and a discussion of leadership and management. These are provided alongside a discussion about their relevance to *nursing* leadership. Analysis of situations in which different styles and approaches can be used, plus the skills and attributes of 'good' leaders, give a grounding for the future chapters. It is important that you have this theoretical background so that you can reflect on the differences between approaches that you will come across in different settings. In addition, the chapter discusses organisational leadership as a complex system – with the aim of providing the 'bigger picture' and so that you can explore the factors that contribute to the success or failure of healthcare organisations. Some key areas of management practices are discussed so that you can see the complexity of a senior leadership role, and can prepare yourself for these areas as you progress through your course. You may well have experience of these and other areas of management from previous roles.

Chapter 3: Policy perspective: Students as the future generations of leaders

Contemporary policy perspectives on nursing leadership are explored. It is acknowledged that policy is a shifting environment – and it is likely (almost certain!) that the policy situation in the UK will have changed since we wrote the book. However, a focus on the history and current situation across the UK nations aims to help you engage meaningfully with the policy landscape. The key aim is to emphasise that understanding and interpreting policy and its impact on the student nurse/newly qualified nurse as a leader is an important aspect of your role. The author makes the case that you should be interested in, and engaged with, policy formation.

Chapter 4: Leadership and inter-professional practice

The context of inter-professional and inter-agency working is described. The landscape of practice continues to evolve, and this chapter is about the shifts that are taking place in nursing and healthcare practice whereby integration is the key agenda – with new approaches coming into place nationally as we write. Leadership of people and organisations across professional boundaries is explored and you are offered the opportunity to look at some of the current changes in the national picture, and how these have (or will) impact on your own role as a leader.

Chapter 5: Leadership from the perspective of the public

Currently, there is a real thrust to ensure that the views of the patient and the public are meaningfully integrated into all aspects of healthcare delivery. The aims of leadership in relation to the public user of care services are explored so that you can think about your own field of practice, and how this aspect of leadership can be further developed.

Chapter 6: Global issues for nursing leadership

Nursing is a global profession and many of the challenges that we face here in the UK are mirrored elsewhere. This chapter discusses the evolving and changing global health-care systems, identifying the challenges for nurse leaders across the globe. The impact of population demographics, the changing focus of health and disease, and their impact on the nurse leaders of the future are explored.

Part Two: Skills, approaches and styles

Chapter 7: The coaching leader

This chapter takes a practical approach to the development of some of the skills for leadership – those of a coaching leader. As part of the approach in the chapter, you are asked to look at your 'self' and at how you can develop a range of skills. The chapter draws on a range of theory, and then homes in on the skills for effective and impact-ful leadership. There is an exploration of emotional intelligence and emotional labour and the application of these important constructs within the context of coaching leadership. In addition, the chapter aims to help you understand yourself as a leader and an individual practitioner. Coaching is, in essence, a two-way process that allows you to explore your input to others as well as to learn more about yourself through a reflective process.

Chapter 8: Networking and leadership

Networking is becoming an ever-more-crucial skill (or skills) for contemporary nursing leaders. This chapter offers arguments which aim to convince you (if you need con-vincing!) of the importance of developing local, national and international networks. Practical examples of how to develop your networks are offered, and the place of social networking is explored. The aim of the chapter is to help you build a picture of your current networks, identify any gaps, and determine how best to increase your networks for particular purposes.

Chapter 9: Preparation for transition to leadership in qualified practice

You may be reading this book as you come towards the end of your pre-registration nurse education, in which case you will be preparing for that transition into qualified practice. This chapter explores the exciting challenges that await you, and the ways in which you can be as well-prepared as possible for leadership and patient care. Some of the key areas under discussion in the chapter are preceptorship, revalidation and ongo-ing development as a leader.

Chapter 10: Harnessing your skills as a future leader: Role models in action

This chapter is based around some semi-structured interviews in which nursing leaders – role models – tell us what leadership is for them, what makes good leadership, and how you can role model those behaviours. They talk about their own leadership journeys so that you can get a feel for the different routes through the profession, and so that you can hopefully feel inspired. Key themes of leadership are drawn from the interviews and summarised so that you can reflect on these themes and their applicability to your own practice. Finally, some light is shone on the need for a good clinical learning environment so that the future leaders of our profession (that's you!) can achieve their potential.

Chapter 11: The student nurse as leader

This is an exciting chapter – you are hearing directly from student nurses. Your voice as a leader is crucial in an era where, for example, attention is focused on raising concerns. The students who contributed to this chapter tell their stories and offer their views on nursing leadership – both reflecting on what they have seen in their clinical placements, and their own experiences of leadership. The aim is to help you reflect on your own leadership styles, giving consideration to what kind of leader you want to be, and appreciating the kind of leader that you might need to be in different situations.

Epilogue: Personal reflections

The two editors have written a short epilogue which tells the story of their own leadership journeys and learning. This is not a chapter which is based on the literature. Rather, it is based on their own personal experiences as nurses, academics and leaders.

PEDAGOGICAL APPROACH: HOW TO USE THE BOOK

We have used a number of different approaches to facilitate your interaction with this book. We expect that you will like some of them, but possibly not all. We are all different! What we hope is that the variety of approaches, with an emphasis on the relevance of the learning to your own practice as a student nurse and leader, will help you to think critically about the theory and enable you to make changes (where you want to) to the way you do things. The book also comes with a companion website (https://study.sagepub.com/taylor), with additional resources to help you learn – including video interviews with nurse leaders and students explaining their experiences of leadership. Below we provide an overview of the approaches we have used, and suggest how these might be useful to you as you dip into and out of the book. We think that one of the most important aspects of this volume is that we have offered insights into 'real-life' practice – through vignettes, research findings, and discussion with students and nurse leaders, both in the book and in the videos on the companion website – so that you can really start to think about how the learning can impact on your own practice.

Chapter learning outcomes

...letion of this chapter you will be able to:

...lore the traits and characteristics of key nursing leaders, and
...uence and legacy.
...amine the nurse as a leader and active participant in an ever-
...veloping system of healthcare.
...cognise the importance of developing leadership skills from th...
...r nurse education and plan how you will develop those skills...

Key concepts

...text of nursing, leadership, trait theories, student...

Chapter learning outcomes
We have provided these at the start of every chapter so that you are clear about what its focus is, and what you might expect to get out of engaging with the theory and the activities.

...t be able to...

...d characteristics of key nursing lead...
...gacy.
...urse as a leader and active participant in an ev...
...ystem of healthcare.
...the importance of developing leadership skills from the
...e education and plan how you will develop those skills.

Key concepts

...ontext of nursing, leadership, trait theories, student as leader

...ION

...is chapter is to offer you an overview of the history
...nship to the current context of nursing and h...
...hread that runs throughout this book – th...
...and the other chapter authors, are...
...le in the leadership of...

Key concepts
A list of key words or phrases gives you an 'at a glance' overview of the main areas under discussion in that chapter.

Activity 1.1

...sing leaders discussed in this chapter
...raits in their approaches to leadership. Co...
...d leader.
...ts of their legacy that you think are relevant t...

...up with words such as passion, visi...
...le model or expert. You may ha...
...re to you. Keep hold of...
...ding on le...

Activities
These are usually reflective in nature and offer you a chance to think about the theory, about your practice, and about yourself as a leader - aiming to facilitate critical thinking and potentially identifying areas where you might want to make changes to the way you do things.

Case study 3.1: Safe Sta...

...f years prior to the founding of the Sa...
...urse staffing levels were dropping. In 20...
stretched. Under-resourced (Buchan and S...
...the workforce and concluding that:

...scenarios in NHS England strongly point to t...
...ses over the next five to 10 years. (Bucha...

...e RCN and the Council of Deans of ...
...urse education places were stori...
...nurses. These reports and ...
...for the NHS in Engl...

Case studies and examples from research
Real-life examples – based on evidence – are
offered as a way of ensuring that you appreciate
the evidence-base for leadership theory and
how it is applied in practice. They illustrate the
concepts and link to the theory that the authors
discuss within the chapters.

Vignettes
We have worked with students and nurse
leaders to include their voices in vignettes
that bring to life the theory and represent
the differing perspectives that exist around
leadership. There are also video interviews on
the companion website for the book (https://
study.sagepub.com/taylor).

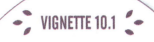

VIGNETTE 10.1

...MBE, Consultant Nurse Cornerstone He...

...e at Cornerstone Health in England. I have ...
...rking in both community learning disabili...
...nursing career within an inpatient learn...
...unity. That's where the bulk of my ...
...s a clinical nurse specialist with l...

...ity of Southampt...

Information box 2.3: Th...

The role of the NHS Board is to:

- Be collectively responsible for
  the success of the organisatio...
  affairs.
- Provide active leadership of the
  effective controls which enable...
- Set the organisation's strateg...
  human resources are in plac...
  review management perfor...
- Set the organisation's ...
  to patients, the loca...

Information boxes
Key pieces of information are provided and
defined within the chapters.

SUMMARY

Some key points from this chapt...

- The skills of listening, reflec
  nursing care.
- The use of a structured coachi
  interactions with patients, sta
- Not to over-emphasise the
  a skill that requires practi

ER RESC

Summaries
End of chapter summaries can be used for quick
reference or revision of key points.

Further resources
The authors have identified further sources
of information that you may wish to access to
deepen your understanding and help you in
assignments. Alongside the book itself, resources
are available on the companion website (https://
study.sagepub.com/taylor) and include links to
useful journal articles, other websites, books,
tools and templates.

...eractions with p...
Not to over-emphasise
a skill that requires practic

FURTHER RESOURCES

Kline, N. (2009) *More Time to Think*. Le
This book provides a further expansion
source for developing your skills.

To access further resources related
https://study.sagepub.com/taylor

...GES

REFLECTION

It is recommended that you come to this book (as to all of your learning) with the aim of critically reflecting on both the theory and your practice. A short overview of an approach to reflection is therefore provided in the box below for you to use as a starting point and to remind you of this key skill.

Reflection for learning

You are asked to undertake reflective exercises within this text. The aim of these exercises will vary, but overall we hope that the act of reflection will facilitate a deeper understanding of the key concepts and ideas that are being explored.

In the context of the learning that you will undertake as you engage with the activities in the book, we have defined reflection as a process that involves six stages based on Gibbs' reflective cycle (Gibbs, 1988):

1. Review the theories and concepts addressed within the activity.
2. Describe the learning gained from the activity.

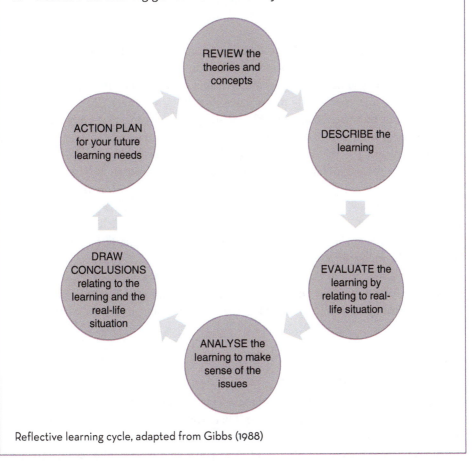

Reflective learning cycle, adapted from Gibbs (1988)

3.   Evaluate the learning by relating it to a real-life situation (for example a practice situation, a learning situation in the university, the findings from a research article).
4.   Analyse the learning so as to make sense of the issues you are exploring.
5.   Come to a conclusion relating to the learning/real-life situation.
6.   Action plan for your future learning needs.

This brief overview gives you a basic framework that you can apply as you do some of the activities in this book. We are sure that you will be actively reflecting as part of your overall learning process, so this won't be news for you! We do think that it is worth saying that the development of rigorous reflective skills is a lifelong process – we are still working on this and finding that as we progress through our careers the value of reflective activity continues to inform our own practices.

WHAT SORT OF BENEFITS DOES THIS BOOK AIM TO BRING TO YOU?

The situation in nursing and healthcare is that change is happening on a daily basis across all services, that there is a strong focus on nursing leadership within all these changes, and that you need to be prepared to stand up and be counted as a leader in your own right. We don't necessarily mean that you will want to be a Chief Nurse (though why not?!), but that you are accountable for all that you do and that every day you have amazing opportunities to make big and small differences to people's lives. This is a huge responsibility and one that requires the development of leadership attributes and skills. As we said at the beginning of this introduction, we passionately believe that you as a student nurse are well-placed to make significant differences to care through your own personal leadership – whether that is by identifying and highlighting concerns, through the development of innovations in practice, or through role modelling in which others see just how nursing should be practised. How exciting to be part of a profession where you can make such a difference!

We go back briefly to the overall objectives for the book – just to unpick these a bit more in readiness for what we explore within the chapters, and so that you can think about how your learning in university and clinical practice can prepare you for what lies ahead.

1. To develop your understanding of theories of leadership and management in healthcare practice

The theoretical basis of leadership and management is crucial to your developing understanding of your own leadership practice. There are multiple books and articles on these topics, as well as websites with excellent information and perspectives. This book aims to provide a broad overview, pointing you towards other resources, and offering a particular perspective – that of *you* at the centre of the learning so that when you go out into your clinical placements you will consciously develop your leadership skills and attributes.

2. To appreciate your role as a leader and a student nurse and how you can impact positively on practice

Linked to what we have just said, we are certain that the greater the critical mass of good role models for leadership at all levels within an organisation, the greater the capacity for excellent care. We show how good leadership is integrally tied to care, compassion and other attributes which have the patient at the centre of care. The exciting part is, as we say, that you can make a difference every day.

3. To apply knowledge of, and skills in, leadership to practice

We have taken a theoretical stance throughout the book as we see evidence-based practice for leadership in the same way that we would see evidence-based practice for the management of particular healthcare needs as vital. What we have done is offer practical situations that enable you to think about that theoretical underpinning in real-life situations. We think that this will help you to take the learning into your own practice so that you can apply these skills in your own everyday practice.

4. To value how your role as a leader can impact positively on the care of service users, carers and relatives, as well as how you can be a role model for colleagues.

Have you thought of yourself as a role model? You may well have, and that's a great thing. We ourselves continually strive to be role models, knowing that we always need to do better – but owning up to it when we make mistakes. What we know is that by striving to be a role model, by working with integrity and strong values, you can make a difference to the team you are working with, and to the care of patients and others.

SUMMARY

This chapter has provided you with an overview of the rationale for our particular approach to the creation of a textbook on leadership for nursing. As you can see, we are passionate about student nurses as leaders and truly believe that *you* can make a difference to healthcare practice through the positive use of your leadership knowledge and skills, and leadership style.

Some key points from this chapter include:

- Leadership is vital for the further development of healthcare practice.
- Student nurses need to develop their leadership skills from the moment they commence their academic programme of study.

- This book is designed to help you in your leadership journey and can be used throughout your university programme.
- Finally, self-awareness, the ability to reflect, eagerness to learn, and the aspiration to be a compassionate care giver, are all equally important contributing attributes of a leader.

FURTHER RESOURCES

For the other chapters, the authors have offered a number of key texts or websites which they feel will enable you to delve more deeply into the theory and into the application of that theory in practice. For the purposes of this introduction, we suggest that you simply revisit literature on reflection so that you feel fully prepared to engage with the learning in this book. We have already offered a summary of reflection based on Gibbs' work, but you may have other literature that you prefer to access. Go ahead and choose whatever works best for you.

 To watch Ruth and Brian discussing the origins, key messages and features of the book, as well as giving you tips on how to be a good leader, please visit the companion website at https://study. sagepub.com/taylor

REFERENCES

Department of Health (2010) *Front Line Care: The Future of Nursing and Midwifery in England.* Report of the Prime Minister's Commission on the Future of Nursing and Midwifery in England. London: The Stationery Office.

Department of Health (2013) *Report of the Mid Staffordshire NHS Foundation Trust Public Inquiry.* Chair Robert Francis QC. London: The Stationery Office.

Gibbs, G. (1988). *Learning by Doing: A Guide to Teaching and Learning Methods.* London: Further Education Unit.

Health Education England (2015) *Raising the Bar. Shape of Caring: A Review of the Future Education and Training of Registered Nurses and Healthcare Assistants.* London: Health Education England and Nursing and Midwifery Council.

Nursing and Midwifery Council (2010) *Standards for Pre-registration Nursing Education.* London: NMC.

Nursing and Midwifery Council (2015) *The Code: Professional Standards of Practice and Behaviour for Nurses and Midwives.* London: NMC.

Scottish Government (2014) *The Vale of Leven Hospital Inquiry Report.* Chair The Rt Hon. Lord MacLean. Scottish Government: Crown.

Taylor, R. (Ed.) (2012) *The Essentials of Nursing and Healthcare Research.* London: Sage.

PART ONE

KNOWLEDGE AND THEORY

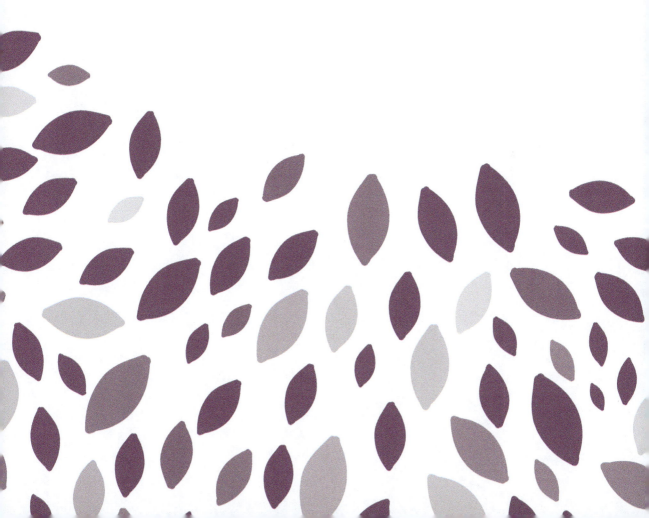

1 THE CONTEXT OF LEADERSHIP IN PRACTICE

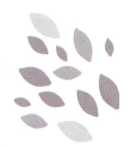

Annette Thomas-Gregory

Chapter learning outcomes

On completion of this chapter you will be able to:

- Explore the traits and characteristics of key nursing leaders, and analyse their influence and legacy.
- Examine the nurse as a leader and active participant in an ever-changing and developing system of healthcare.
- Recognise the importance of developing leadership skills from the beginning of your nurse education and plan how you will develop those skills.

Key concepts

Historical context of nursing, leadership, trait theories, student as leader

INTRODUCTION

The purpose of this chapter is to offer you an overview of the history of nursing leadership and its relationship to the current context of nursing and healthcare practice. Linked to this is the thread that runs throughout this book – the importance of the student nurse as a leader. I, and the other chapter authors, are making the case that as a student nurse you have a key role in the leadership of nursing practice. You may not recognise this just now – after all, you may be a new first year student and may not see that leadership is part of what you do at present. However, I hope to shift your perspective if that is needed, and help you to see how you *are* a leader – sometimes in small everyday ways, and sometimes in relation to the big issues that are current within our healthcare system. The focus on leadership is important in terms of ensuring that all staff can advocate for patients and raise an alarm if the care is not as good as it should be; and that every nurse whatever their role, context of care or experience is able to take a lead in ensuring that patients get the best quality of care.

By taking you through a short journey of leadership in nursing, I aim to emphasise some of the characteristics and attributes that leaders need in nursing practice, and also acknowledge that the context of nursing practice has shifted, and continues to shift, with an associated impact on nursing leadership.

BACKGROUND: HISTORICAL OVERVIEW OF NURSING LEADERS

This section provides a summary of a number of key nursing leaders in history, and offers a perspective on some of their traits and characteristics. It is a fact that historically nursing was a female-dominated profession. However, things are changing and there are now many examples of male nurses in leadership positions.

Florence Nightingale is seen as the founder of modern nursing. She led nursing in the Crimean War and founded a school of nursing at St Thomas' Hospital in London in the late 19th century. Part of her legacy is that she developed professional nursing roles, and emphasised the need for nursing leadership. She advocated that the success of nursing depended on (quoted in Helmstadter, 1997: 1039):

> The authority and discipline over all the women of a trained lady superintendent who is also matron of the hospital, and who is herself the best nurse in the hospital, the example and the leader of her nurses in all that she wishes her nurses to be.

The position of the matron was to become critical to the reform and modernisation of the hospital system of nursing. However, despite this innovation, in most hospitals issues regarding the nature of nursing, the training of nurses, and recruitment of nurses were referred to the medical committee for approval (Wildman and Hewison, 2009). Florence Nightingale was viewed as an early embodiment of leadership in nursing. She wielded personal power and influenced policy but according to some she did little to discourage this subservience to medicine. Perhaps you might feel that the traits/characteristics that she exhibited included a vision for nursing practice, the determination and motivation to achieve her vision, and the courage to do what she thought would improve nursing practice. You may however have other ideas about the kind of leader that Nightingale was.

Ethel Bedford Fenwick (1857–1947) was a distinguished contemporary of Florence Nightingale. She worked hard and showed an aptitude for management, attracting the attention of people in positions of influence, and she moved to St Bartholomew's Hospital in London as matron at the age of 24. She aspired to train nurses and improve the standards of nursing. Throughout her career she campaigned for better conditions for nursing staff. Perhaps most notable of all was her campaign for nurses to have professional independence, and between 1887 and 1899 she campaigned for the registration of nurses and developed the British Nurses Association (BNA) which would protect their interests and offer them registration. Bedford Fenwick also founded the International Council of Nurses (ICN) to promote co-operation between nurses of all countries and to provide them with opportunities to meet and discuss professional issues – this to many was her greatest achievement. Again, you might feel that Bedford Fenwick displayed traits or characteristics such as vision, influencing skills, determination and dedication to the vision.

Another notable nurse leader was Mary Seacole who was born in Jamaica in 1805, the daughter of a black mother and a white Scottish father. Mary was also a contemporary of Florence Nightingale, and volunteered to go to the Crimea with the Nightingale nurses. She felt that her experiences of treating soldiers in Panama would be useful to the nurses in the Crimea where similar conditions prevailed. Mary was to be disappointed. She was rejected because of her age and colour. However she refused to give up and decided to travel to the Crimea on her own and set up her 'British Hotel' where sick soldiers could convalesce. Unlike Florence Nightingale, Mary Seacole received little fame or notoriety for her role in the Crimean war. Following the war she returned home penniless and destitute having funded her travel and work from her own pocket. When considering Seacole's leadership characteristics, words that may come to mind may include courage, vision and determination.

Virginia Henderson (1896–1996) attended an army school of nursing in Washington DC and went on to a teacher training college in Columbia University graduating with a Master's in nursing education. In 1955 she co-authored the *Textbook of the Principles and Practice of Nursing* (Harmer and Henderson, 1955). She advocated a new and distinctive philosophical model or approach towards nursing practice, which emphasised independence. Perhaps her leadership characteristics or traits could be described as visionary, having expertise and being collaborative. Henderson's work is most famously identified by her belief that:

> The unique function of the nurse is to assist the individual, sick or well, in the performance of those activities contributing to health or its recovery (or to peaceful death) that he would perform unaided if he had the necessary strength, will or knowledge, and to do this in such a way as to help him gain independence as rapidly as possible. (Harmer and Henderson, 1955, in Klainberg, 2010: 35)

The first practising Muslim nurse, according to many Islamic scholars, was Rufaidah Al-Islamiah. When the Prophet Mohammad went with his followers to fight the first battle against their enemies a group of Muslim women, including Al-Islamiah, participated by providing moral support and looking after the wounded soldiers (Al-Rifai, 1996). After they won the battle Al-Islamiah continued to provide her services to sick people, believing that nursing was an art required by people during days of peace and war. Perhaps Al-Islamiah's leadership characteristics or traits included compassion, vision and determination?

As you can maybe see from these accounts, the narrative around nursing leadership tends towards descriptions of great people with particular traits. The trait theories are some of the oldest theories on leadership; they are also referred to as 'Great Man theories', suggesting that an individual is born a great leader. These are explored in more depth in Chapter 2.

Florence Nightingale, Ethel Bedford Fenwick, Mary Seacole, Virginia Henderson and Rufaidah Al-Islamiah are notable examples of illustrious nurses with amazing leadership skills. Perhaps it is their enduring legacy that makes them great leaders? Or their ability to challenge the status quo? You may think it relates to their courage to take risks and not give up, and their passion and integrity? These are all areas worthy of discussion and consideration and are very relevant to current issues in nursing and healthcare where the need for leadership that demonstrates courage, integrity, a common mission, commitment and care is essential to the quality of healthcare.

Activity 1.1

Reflect on the nursing leaders discussed in this chapter. Make a list of the characteristics or traits in their approaches to leadership. Consider what you think makes them a good leader.

Are there aspects of their legacy that you think are relevant to you as a developing nursing leader?

You may have come up with words such as passion, vision, caring, determination, resilience, commitment, role model or expert. You may have come up with some other words or phrases that mean more to you. Keep hold of these words or phrases and consider them as you continue your reading on leadership in nursing. You might change your view or wish to add more to your list of characteristics and traits.

There are numerous contemporary examples of nursing leaders who are well-known for different reasons. Some of these include the three individuals described below.

As a student nurse Molly Case caused a sensation at the RCN Congress in 2013. As well as being a student nurse at the time, she is also a spoken word artist. Her poem demonstrated an understanding of the issues affecting nursing as a profession at the time, and demonstrated that student nurses could speak out and make a difference. Here is the link to the video of that event: www.youtube.com/watch?v=XOCda6OiYpg. More is written about her in Chapter 11.

David Benton is the Chief Executive of the International Council of Nurses (http://leadership.icn.ch/gnli/david-benton). If you read his profile you can see that he has had a varied career crossing practice, management and policy.

Matthew Hodson MBE was named *Nursing Standard* Nurse of the Year in 2013 for his contribution to respiratory nursing. He is seen as an inspiration to many and someone who continues to contribute to nursing practice in ways that make positive differences to the patient experience.

Activity 1.2

You have a list of words or phrases from Activity 1.1. Spend some time thinking about the nursing leaders that you have met on clinical placement.

- What characteristics or traits stand out for you in these leaders?
- Are these positive or negative in your view?

THE DEVELOPMENT OF THE POLICY CONTEXT ACROSS THE UK

Leadership cannot occur within a vacuum – context is essential. It is important to have an understanding of UK health policy in order to contextualise the role of nursing leadership in practice. Nurses working in the NHS in the 1980s would have performed very different roles and faced different challenges from those working in the early years of the new millennium. You will witness great changes in the management and context of care as you progress through your course and your subsequent career. In this section I explore some aspects of the historical political context that have influenced the shape of care in the UK and consider policy changes that have and will influence the manner in which nurses practise and the implications for leadership in practice. These issues are explored in greater depth in Chapter 3.

It took a number of factors to establish registration for all trained nurses. Following World War One (1914–1918) trained nurses sought to distance themselves from the large numbers of untrained nurses that had helped to care for the huge number of casualties in the war (Williamson et al., 2008). This, alongside the campaigns by suffragettes for equal votes for women, brought about the political context needed to allow the registration of nurses to be taken seriously. In 1916 the Royal College of Nursing was founded and in 1919 the Nurses Registration Act was passed in parliament which established the General Nursing Council (GNC) register for nurses. However, following a lengthy period of time, it was recognised that the supply of registered nurses could not meet the demand in practice and many hospitals were recruiting assistants to help the registered nurses. In 1943 it was agreed that these 'assistant nurses' would be allowed onto the GNC register if they had completed two years of training. This development in nursing was viewed by some as a significant move towards a two-tiered profession with registered nurses being seen as the professional leaders of nursing and the assistants being capable followers.

In 1979, the Nurses, Midwives and Health Visitors Act followed recommendations by the Briggs Committee (Department of Health and Social Security, 1972) and transformed the GNC into the more powerful United Kingdom Central Council for

Nursing, Midwifery and Health Visiting (UKCC). This new organisation had similar responsibilities to the GNC in that it approved training institutions, regulated standards of training and conduct and regulated entry to the register. This regulatory body was further transformed in 2002 when it became the Nursing and Midwifery Council (NMC), our current statutory regulatory body. The NMC regulates nurses and midwives in the UK and exists to protect the public (NMC, 2015). It sets the standards for education and training.

The origins of nurse education programmes in the higher education sector can also be traced back to the early 1970s and the report of the Committee of Nursing (Department of Health and Social Security, 1972). This report presented a strong indictment of the need for nursing in the NHS to be better recognised and supported, and argued for root and branch reform focusing particularly on the separation of service from education (Kitson, 2001). In 1984 all but 2% of nurse training was delivered within the NHS. However, following the UKCC Project 2000 review, 100% of nurse training was to be relocated into higher education. Following years of management by district health authorities in the NHS, nurse education was removed financially, legally and structurally from the NHS, with the closure of traditional hospital-based schools of nursing (Watson and Thompson, 2004).

The move into higher education has many benefits for nursing and reflects the development of the profession. In 2009 the then Health Minister Ann Keen announced that all nurses entering training would undertake degree-level education so as to increase their skills (e.g. in relation to analysis and autonomy of practice) (*Guardian*, 2009). This notion challenged misconceptions that nursing was a vocational, non-academic occupation for which a degree was unnecessary. In a world of rapidly changing and increasingly complex healthcare, it is necessary that nurses are equipped with the knowledge and skills to deliver compassionate care within very different contexts and roles (McGrory, 2009).

There were concurrent changes within healthcare delivery. The National Health Service (NHS), established in 1948, had been recognised as one of the largest organisations in Europe and one of the best health services in the world. The founders of the NHS believed that a civilised society should ensure that everyone had equal access to healthcare, and therefore the NHS was developed along the following principles (Rivett, 2007):

- The NHS would be financed virtually 100% through taxation – therefore both rich and poor would pay in proportion to their means.
- Everyone would be eligible for care.
- Healthcare would be free at the point of need.

Many of the current issues and tensions that affect the management and administration of the modern NHS emerged quite soon after it was established. It became clear that public expectations were high and that funding for such an enterprise would be a never-ending concern. Aneurin Bevin, the principal architect of the NHS, foresaw this issue and is quoted in Rivett (2007):

We shall never have all we need. Expectations will always exceed capacity. The service must always be changing, growing and improving – it must always appear inadequate.

During the 1980s and 1990s there became an increasing urgency for health service reform and action to manage the growing number of issues arising related to healthcare in the UK. The NHS *Priorities and Planning Guidance* (DH, 1997) stated that:

With necessarily limited financial and management resources, the fundamental challenge for managers and professionals is to strike a balance between resolving immediate and conflicting pressures and to continue to make good progress in development areas.

In 1998 the NHS celebrated 50 years of healthcare for all. Whilst staff, patients and the public were encouraged to look back at this remarkable achievement, attention was focused on putting into action one of the biggest programmes of change that the NHS had ever witnessed: placing patients at the centre of the NHS. The publication of *The NHS Plan* (DH, 2000) set out a series of comprehensive plans to transform the NHS into a health service fit for the 21st century, and it promised:

- More hospitals and beds.
- More doctors and nurses.
- Shorter waiting times for hospital and GP appointments.
- Cleaner wards and better food in hospitals.
- Improved care for the elderly.
- Tougher standards for NHS organisations and rewards for the best.
- Greater power and more information for patients and the public.

Much has changed since *The NHS Plan* was first published, but every development and initiative since had its roots in the core vision of creating a patient-led health service. This vision was that NHS services would be built upon the needs and preferences of patients rather than dictated by barriers in the system, and between professional groups. It depended upon improvements in communication and service structure so that wherever possible care would take place where it was convenient to patients – close to home in the community setting. This policy drive is still unfolding, but a number of initiatives and policy documents have demonstrated that the vision is sustained and developing momentum despite political changes.

As you have probably seen when you have been in your practice areas, the NHS across the UK is dealing with an increasingly complex array of health and social care needs. Alongside these challenges, staff need to be responsive to different cultural norms, values, beliefs and lifestyles and different healthcare needs. You are probably conscious of an increasingly media-aware and informed public – a good thing, but that can some-times bring its own challenges. The overall picture is that people are living longer with

increasingly complex long-term health conditions alongside increasingly high expectations of healthcare services. Nursing is amongst the many healthcare disciplines that
is, and will be, increasingly challenged to respond to the changing needs of the public.
Chapter 3 provides a more in-depth view of policy for healthcare and nursing across the
UK. You will find many similarities and some differences in direction and vision. For the
purposes of this chapter, I have focused on a small number of illustrative policies – but
feel free to access those most relevant to your context. For example, *High Quality Care for
All* (DH, 2008: 25–30) identified six areas of challenge for the NHS in the 21st century:

- Rising expectations.
- Demand driven by demographics.
- The information society.
- Advances in treatment.
- The changing nature of disease.
- The changing nature of the health workplace.

With these challenges in mind the key areas that are changing for nurses and other
healthcare practitioners include the shift towards a primary care led NHS, the development of new organisations such as social enterprises (businesses that can bid for funds,
deliver services and are driven by social benefit) and an increase in technology-based
care. The one thing that doesn't change is the limitation in terms of financial means
to satisfy everyone, and most healthcare practitioners will have experienced different
forms of rationing/cuts in healthcare expenditure. For nursing, the changes present not
only challenges but also opportunities, including the change to an all-graduate profession, reforms in career structure, flexible roles, and emerging roles that require nurses
to be increasingly independent, autonomous and able to co-ordinate care. In order to
achieve high quality care within this ever-changing context, nurses need to demonstrate
leadership qualities such as integrity, courage, commitment, compassion, competence
and care – those qualities that are espoused by the *NHS Constitution* (DH, 2009) and
our NMC *Code of Conduct* (2015).

Activity 1.3

- Reflect on how the changes in the organisation of the NHS are likely to impact
  upon future roles for nurses.
- What are the key challenges for nurses who are leading currently and in the
  future?

You may have thought about some of the new roles emerging in practice, such
as Advanced Nurse Practitioners and Nurse Consultants – roles that may have been
around for some time, but which are evolving as the context of healthcare delivery

changes. Some of these roles are developing because there is a need for nurses to acquire advanced knowledge and practice skills, such as prescribing, diagnostic and clinical decision-making skills in a range of settings. I would imagine that one of the challenges that you considered was what sort of education and training these nurses would need so that they are properly prepared to perform these expanded roles and how they would be supported in their development. You might wish to read more in *The Shape of Caring: A Review of the Future Education and Training of Registered Nurses and Care Assistants* (Health Education England, 2015).

LEADERSHIP PREPARATION AND THE STUDENT NURSE AS A DEVELOPING LEADER

The scale of the changes affecting all healthcare practitioners in the UK might be viewed as relentless and may create negative feelings in some people. Others might consider the changes as opening opportunities, and feel energised by the evolving healthcare context. For some it might seem that the changes in the NHS are the concern of senior figures and outside the remit of junior nurses. In this section I would like to emphasise how important it is that all nurses understand the health service reconfiguration and are actively engaged in leading healthcare reform. In short the student nurses of today are the leaders of tomorrow and need to be developing aspects of both clinical and political leadership throughout their education, including sustaining their moral purpose, enthusiasm, energy and hope, and understanding the infrastructure and changes occurring within the NHS (Fullan, 2001). An excellent animation of the new NHS in England is available at the King's Fund and it may help to point you to areas that you need to investigate further: www.kingsfund.org.uk/projects/nhs-65/alternative-guide-new-nhs-england. Similarly, the following websites provide overviews of the structure of the NHS in the rest of the UK: www.ournhsscotland.com/our-nhs/nhsscotland-how-it-works, www.wales.nhs.uk/nhswalesaboutus/structure, www.dhsspsni.gov.uk/topics.

Activity 1.4

- Reflect on your own degree programme: what aspects of leadership and management have you been taught to date?
- Analyse this knowledge and identify how you might further develop your own leadership skills.

You might have reflected on a number of taught sessions on leadership and management and/or role transition. Maybe you have a module that covers issues related to developing leadership skills within your final year as a student? Curtis et al. (2011)

suggest that leadership is an essential part of nursing practice and should be threaded longitudinally through the curriculum and practice learning. Recent studies (Cummings et al., 2008; Hughes et al., 2006) have indicated that personality traits, experience and age also influence the ability to lead in clinical practice, and, most importantly, where leadership is taught and integrated into nursing it has a positive impact upon nursing practice.

As you will know, the NMC (2010) publish the standards for pre-registration nurse education. These take the form of a developmental framework for all fields of nursing and include:

- Professional values.
- Communication and interpersonal skills.
- Nursing practice and decision-making.
- Leadership, management and team working.

In relation to 'leadership, management and team working', the standards state that nurses must *act as change agents* and provide leadership through quality improvement and service development to enhance people's wellbeing and experiences of healthcare. They must *systematically evaluate care* and ensure that they and others use the findings to help improve people's experience and care outcomes and shape future services. In addition, nurses must be able to *identify priorities and manage time and resources* effectively to ensure the quality of care is maintained or enhanced. They must *be self-aware* and recognise how their own values, principles and assumptions may affect their practice. They must maintain their own personal and professional development, learning from experience, through supervision, feedback, reflection and evaluation. They have a responsibility to *facilitate nursing students and others to develop their competence*, using a range of professional and personal development skills. They must also *work independently as well as in teams and work effectively across professional and agency boundaries*.

You might be forgiven if you are wondering how you can develop the necessary knowledge, skills and attitudes to fulfil all of these competencies. However, to reassure you, Bower (2000) claims that the main qualities of a leader are based on a range of skills and attitudes that can be developed by anyone motivated enough to attain them, and claims that there is leadership potential in everyone. As you work your way through this book and engage with some of the activities, you will be able to identify other areas in which you wish to develop and use the tools provided to enable you to do that. One example is provided here to enable you to start reflecting further on aspects of your role as a student nurse and leader – your role as a facilitator of learning.

Depending on what stage you are in your learning, you may already be working with more junior student nurses and will understand (from your own experience) how important it is to facilitate their learning. As you work towards the completion of your course and then subsequently move into newly qualified practice, the need for you to be able to take on a teaching/facilitation role will become more important. Many student nurses start developing skills in mentorship by supporting students in the years below them. Learning in a clinical environment is particularly meaningful where that learning environment enables the student to feel safe, valued and stimulated. Within a learning environment an essential aspect of learning relates to role modelling, therefore it is important that leaders within the environment demonstrate integrity and honesty about their knowledge limits, and curiosity in areas of uncertainty. You may be able to think of examples where you have had to do just that.

Activity 1.5

Think about a mentor who inspired you. Write down the reasons why that mentor had an influence on you. Make a list of how you might incorporate some of those characteristics into your own leadership practice.

Finally, in this section I would like you to think about the characteristics or attributes that you believe should exist in a nursing leader. Remember, you are also a nurse leader, albeit at the beginning of your career. You lead aspects of care on a daily basis when you are in practice – even when you are new to nursing there are times when you, for example, interact with a patient when your mentor is not around. Your role as a student nurse leader is vital in these interactions and your leadership is demonstrated through the use of interpersonal skills, the decisions you take based upon those interactions, and the impact you have on the patient experience in those situations. So as a final exercise for this section, Activity 1.6 aims to pull together the learning from history alongside the NMC leadership, management and team working competencies – to help you develop a personal map for your own development.

Activity 1.6

- Go back to your list of characteristics that you developed for Activity 1.1. Which of these do you want to develop further?
- Now look at the competencies outlined in this section and decide which of these you need to enhance for your own practice.

With these lists, you should now identify the ways in which you can further develop the skills and attributes. Here are some suggestions:

- Use one or more as a focus for your learning in your next clinical placement. Talk to your mentor about this, and develop an action plan for your learning.

(Continued)

(Continued)

- Identify some evidence-based articles through which you can broaden your knowledge and understanding. Construct a mind map or a summary of the learning from the articles and then consider how best to apply the learning in a practice situation.
- Ask one of your peers to discuss one or more of the areas. Find out what you both understand about the topic, and then work together to develop your knowledge-base.

SUMMARY

The key points for your learning in this chapter include:

- Appreciating aspects of the historical development of nursing places the role of the nurse as leader within a context – one that is shifting as the political, health, social and other drivers impact on healthcare practice.
- The NMC leadership, management and team working competencies provide a framework for developing some key aspects of learning as the building blocks for clinical leadership.
- Leadership is built upon a strong sense of moral purpose, hope, passion and resilience – it may be a challenge, but it is exciting to work towards the opportunities that will enable you to develop and sustain these aspects of your professional identity.

FURTHER RESOURCES

Health Education England (2015) *The Shape of Caring: A Review of the Future Education and Training of Registered Nurses and Care Assistants.* [Online] Available at https://hee.nhs.uk/work-programmes/shape-of-caring-review.
This is a relatively recent publication from Health Education England which will give you insight into some of the emerging roles in practice and some of the education and training necessary to prepare nurses for expanded and advanced roles in the context of changes in care delivery.

Lorentzon, M. and Bryant, J. (1997) 'Leadership in British nursing: a historical dimension'. *Journal of Nursing Management*, 5: 271–8.
This article provides a good overview of the historical dimensions of British nursing leadership, linking history to the context of nursing practice at the time.

www.kingsfund.org.uk/projects/nhs-65/alternative-guide-new-nhs-england.
The King's Fund website is an excellent resource for leadership and policy information and critique. As cited earlier in the chapter, the animation on the new NHS provides information in an accessible way. You may want to explore other areas in the King's Fund website and perhaps sign up to their alerts.

 To access further resources related to this chapter, please visit the companion website at https://study.sagepub.com/taylor

REFERENCES

Al-Rifai (1996) *Nursing Workforce Capacity Building in the UAE.* [Online] Available at http://webcache.googleusercontent.com/search?q=cache:iWoBEyqbnbsJ:www.researchgate.net/profile/Sharon_Brownie/publication/259495987_Nursing_Workforce_Capacity_Building_in_the_UAE_Progress_Issues_and_Matters_of_Assessment/links/00b4952c47b257ab01000000.pdf+&cd=5&hl=en&ct=clnk&gl=uk&client=safari. Accessed 15/08/15.

Bower, F.L. (2000) *Nurses Taking the Lead: Personal Qualities of Effective Leadership:* Philadelphia: WB Saunders Company.

Cummings, G., Lee, H. and MacGregor, T. (2008) 'Factors contributing to nursing leadership: a systematic review'. *Journal of Health Service Policy*, 13(4): 240–8.

Curtis, E., De Vries, J. and Sheerin, F. (2011) 'Developing leadership in nursing: exploring core factors'. *British Journal of Nursing*, 20(5): 306–9.

Department of Health and Social Security (1972) *Report of the Committee of Nursing* (The Briggs Report). Cmnd 5715. London: HMSO.

Department of Health (1997) *Priorities and Planning Guidance for the NHS: 1998/99.* Leeds: NHS Executive. [Online] Available at http://webarchive.nationalarchives.gov.uk/+/www.dh.gov.uk/en/Publicationsandstatistics/Publications/PublicationsPolicyAndGuidance/DH_4006170. Accessed 15/05/15.

Department of Health (2000) *The NHS Plan: a Plan for Investment, a Plan for Reform.* London: DH.

Department of Health (2008) *High Quality Care for All: NHS Next Stage Review Final Report.* London: DH.

Department of Health (2009) *The NHS Constitution: The NHS Belongs to Us All.* London: DH.

Fullan, M. (2001) *Leading in a Culture of Change.* San Francisco, CA: John Wiley & Sons, Jossey-Bass.

Guardian (2009, 12 November) 'All new nurses to have degrees from 2013'. [Online] Available at www.theguardian.com/society/2009/nov/12/nurses-nursing-qualifications-degrees-nmc-rcn. Accessed 7/6/2016.

Harmer, B. and Henderson, V. (1955) *Textbook of the Principles and Practice of Nursing.* London: Macmillan.

Health Education England (2015) *The Shape of Caring: A Review of the Future Education and Training of Registered Nurses and Care Assistants.* London: NMC.

Helmstadter, C. (1997) 'Doctors and nurses in the London teaching hospitals: class, gender, religion and professional expertise'. *Nursing History Review*, 5: 161–97.

Hughes, R., Ginnett, R. and Curphy, G. (2006) *Leadership: Enhancing the Lessons of Experience*, 5th edition. Boston, MA: McGraw-Hill.

Kitson, A. (2001) 'Nursing leadership: bringing caring back to the future'. *Quality in Healthcare*, 10(Suppl. 2): ii79–ii84.

Klainberg, M. (2010) *An Historical Overview of Nursing.* In Klainberg, M. and Dirschel, K. (eds), *Today's Nursing Leader: Managing, Succeeding, Excelling.* Sudbury, MA: Jones and Bartlett Publishers.

McGrory, C. (2009) 'Nursing is a professional role'. *British Journal of Nursing*, 18(21): 1288.

Nursing and Midwifery Council (2010) *Standards for Pre-Registration Nursing Education.* London: NMC.

Nursing and Midwifery Council (2015) *Code of Conduct.* [Online] Available at www.nmc.org.uk/globalassets/sitedocuments/nmc-publications/revised-new-nmc-code.pdf. Accessed 15/05/15.

Rivett, G.C. (2007) *National Health Service History*. [Online] Available at www.nhshistory.net/shorthistory.htm. Accessed 15/08/15.

Watson, R. and Thompson, D. (2004) 'The Trojan horse of nurse education'. *Nurse Education Today*, 24: 73–5.

Wildman, S. and Hewison, A. (2009) 'Re-discovering a history of nursing management: from Nightingale to the modern matron'. *International Journal of Nursing Studies*, 46(12): 1650–61. [Online] Available at www.journalofnursingstudies.com/article/S0020-7489(09)00205-3/references. Accessed 18/01/16.

Williamson, G., Jenkinson, T. and Proctor-Childs, T. (2008) *Contexts of Contemporary Nursing*, 2nd edition. Exeter: Learning Matters Ltd.

2 NURSING LEADERSHIP IN ORGANISATIONS

Theory and practice

Alison Crombie and Gayle Garland

Chapter learning outcomes

On completion of this chapter you will be able to:

- Describe the role of theory in the development of leadership and management practice within nursing organisations.
- Identify the key responsibilities and factors that influence individual leadership practice.
- Discuss organisational leadership as a complex system, and explore factors that contribute to success or failure.

Key concepts

Leadership, management, nursing organisations, policy

INTRODUCTION

Management and leadership theories have been developed in an attempt to explain the nature of such skills and attributes, and to guide individuals in their practice of leading and managing. By looking more widely than just the individual's personal characteristics, skills and behaviour, the practice of leadership and management has been continually evolving, and now offers some insight into how you as a student nurse may develop and apply your leadership and management abilities and skills in practice.

This chapter looks at the importance of theory, and analyses the impact this has on the practice of leadership and management in nursing. A particular emphasis is placed on the role of senior leaders within organisations alongside the policy and organisational contexts within which they operate. This emphasis on senior leadership should not detract from the focus of this book – the student nurse as leader – but rather is used as an illustration to help you think through your future vision, aspirations and potential. Threaded throughout this chapter are our thoughts on how you, as a student nurse and leader, can develop your leadership capability and make a difference to practice now as well as in the future.

LEADERSHIP AND MANAGEMENT: DEFINITIONS

You may already be aware of the discourse that surrounds the two terms – leadership and management. As a starting point for this chapter, some overarching definitions are provided with the aim of identifying what is relevant to you as you develop as a leader. Given that the title and focus of this book are leadership, most of what follows relates to leadership theory. However, the differences between leadership and management are not binary, as will hopefully become clearer as the chapter progresses. Both concepts come together as new ways of leadership practice come into being for our evolving healthcare system. It is important to be clear that we are not saying that management is not relevant to nursing practice. On the contrary, there are lots of examples of where management skills are *essential* – for example, a manager will need to manage the budget effectively and ensure that patient 'flow' through the system is effective. However, leadership in this context would relate to the *way* in which these management requirements are handled, communicated and manoeuvred, as you will see as you progress through your learning on your course – both in university and in practice.

Management can be described as the processes that enable things to get done through a formal role – usually someone who has been given authority within an organisation to take forward particular responsibilities. A manager of a department will have responsibility for the budget, staffing and resources, and the overall achievement of organisational targets or goals. Management of a particular situation or a department is usually better achieved where leadership skills are utilised, as we hope you will see.

Stanley (2009: 22) has defined leadership in these terms:

> Leadership is seen in terms of unifying people around values and then constructing the social world for others around those values and helping people to get through change.

Taylor (2009) suggests that this 'definition' encapsulates some of the core concepts associated with leadership: values, facilitation of change, interpersonal skills and engagement with 'followers'. As you can probably already see, leadership is not one thing or one approach – it is a concept that can be broadly defined as we have here, and one which depends on the particular approach or perspective that the leader comes from. It perhaps goes without saying that leaders can't exist without followers. Our assertion is that, depending on the context, you will as a student nurse sometimes be acting in a leadership role, and will sometimes be acting in a follower role.

The chapter goes on to discuss some core leadership theories: Great Man, trait, situational/contingency, transactional and transformational. The purpose of the discussion in this chapter is to set the scene and provide a basis from which you can explore these theories further and start to consider your own leadership style as it is currently, and give some thought to how you would like to develop as a leader.

PERSONAL LEADERSHIP JOURNEY: EVER-PRESENT LEADERSHIP

We are sure that you would agree that leadership is a topic that is important to students, not only because it is a competency set by the Nursing and Midwifery Council (NMC) to be achieved in order to become registered, but because it is also an essential set of skills for safe and effective care (NMC, 2010). Leadership as a concept has evolved and developed over time, though the attempt to develop theory to explain leadership is relatively recent. Historians in the 19th century sought to understand why a few individuals have had such a disproportionate effect on history. Thomas Carlyle, a Scottish writer, published a book called *On Heroes, Hero Worship and the Heroic in History* (1841) in which he suggested that the important turning points in history can be largely explained by the impact of 'great men', who had superior wisdom, skills, intelligence or charisma. His book described the lives of well-known heroes of the past such as Shakespeare and Napoleon as support for his idea and became known as the *Great Man Theory*. It influenced thinking from that point forward and in particular led to the development of the trait theories of leadership.

There were critics of the Great Man theory, particularly among social scientists. For example, Herbert Spencer (1896) argued that great men were created by their circumstances and the society they lived in. He suggested that it was a complex combination of factors including their race, status in society, their education, and connection to important events that led to the greatness they achieved. Whether or not you agree with the Great Man theory (men creating history) or the critics (society creating great men), it is clear that nursing as a profession has had its share of what we will call 'Great Nurses' (see Chapter 1).

The study of great leaders gave rise to the next evolution of leadership thinking called the *Trait Theory* of leadership. This theory was underpinned by the idea that great leaders shared a number of traits or personal characteristics that enabled them to have impact as a leader; if people could develop the traits and skills of great leaders, they could become more effective at leading.

One of the problems with trait leadership as an approach to understanding and developing people as leaders is that a great many traits were identified – so many in fact that the list became little more than a set of virtuous attributes. Some traits that made the list, such as being dominant, assertive and ambitious, were characteristic of only some effective leaders (in business and industry perhaps) but arguably not typical of leaders in other situations or fields. There was a growing recognition that whilst traits and skills provide a foundation for leadership, it is the leader's *actions* that create results. This recognition gave rise to the next set of leadership theories, classed together as behavioural theories of leadership.

Behavioural Theories of leadership were devised from the study of what successful leaders *do*: how they behave in response to the challenges they face and to achieve the outcomes they want. One of the earliest theorists to write about leadership behaviour was Max Weber (1905) who discussed two types of leader: the bureaucratic leader and the charismatic leader. The bureaucratic leader was one who took a structured approach to leading, following procedure to ensure that things were done properly and safely. He suggested this was the best method of managing large organisations such as banks, hospitals and universities where quality and safety were hugely important aspects of the organisation. The charismatic leadership approach was one where the leader used energy and enthusiasm to inspire people, most suited in his view to organisations in which design and innovation were needed. Weber and colleagues described three additional behavioural styles: autocratic (leading by a show of power and authority); democratic (leading by involving others); and laissez-faire (leading by giving authority to others) (Taylor, 2009).

Early behavioural theories of leadership were important in developing the idea that a range of different leadership actions can be effective depending on the people you lead and the situation you find yourself in. Most people would agree that autocratic leadership is most effective in an emergency situation where power and authority are exercised by the leader. It would be ineffective to hold a staff meeting (democratic leadership) to determine who should call the fire services during a fire emergency. Similarly, we would argue that it is equally inappropriate to use a laissez-faire leadership style to manage an outbreak of a viral infection on a ward. These insights gave rise to the next wave of leadership theories called contingency or situational leadership theories.

Contingency or *Situational* leadership theories suggest that the most effective leadership style is the one that takes into consideration the situation, the follower and the task. Fieldler (1967) became recognised as one of the pioneers of this way of thinking, but perhaps the best known of these theories is Situational Leadership© theory by Hersey and Blanchard (1969) which suggested that leaders should use one of four styles: the telling style for situations in which the followers are reluctant and unskilled; the selling style when followers are willing but lack skill; the participating style when followers are competent but lack in confidence; and the delegating style when followers are competent, experienced and willing.

Activity 2.1

Think of an individual you consider to be a recognised leader. What makes them a good leader? Write a short tribute to that person for a blog or online profile, considering their traits, behaviours and situations they have encountered. This should help you to really think about what you most value in the leaders that you are connected to.

Transactional and *Transformational* leadership are more recent theoretical approaches and relate very much to the culture of a work environment. Transactional leadership could be described as being closer to the management end of a spectrum of leadership approaches, whereas transformational leadership focuses on the relationships within the leader/follower context. Table 2.1 offers a summary of the differences between the two approaches.

Linked particularly to transformational leadership, Stanley's *Congruent* leadership (which is where we started the discussion on leadership in this chapter) is hugely important for nursing practice as you may agree that being able to practise as a leader in ways that are *congruent* with your values is important in the context of healthcare practice.

Table 2.1   Transactional and transformational leadership (taken from Taylor, 2009, originally Covey, 1992)

Transactional theories	Transformational theories
Builds on people's need to get a job done and make a living	Builds on people's need for meaning
Is preoccupied with power, position, politics and perks	Is preoccupied with purposes and values, morals and ethics
Is mired in daily affairs	Transcends daily affairs
Is short-term and hard data orientated	Is orientated towards long-term goals without compromising human values and principles
Focuses on tactical issues	Focuses more on mission and strategies
Relies on human relations to lubricate human interactions	Releases human potential identifying and developing new talent
Follows and fulfils role expectations by striving to work effectively within current systems	Designs and redesigns jobs to make them meaningful and challenging
Supports structures and systems that reinforce the bottom line, maximise efficiency and guarantee short-term profits	Aligns internal structures and systems to reinforce values and goals

LEADERSHIP IN NURSING

The modern concept of leadership and management in nursing practice draws to some extent on the theories that have emerged in recent decades. Scientific management can be seen in the development of policies and procedures to guide practice in nursing and many other health professions. Quality improvement strategies such as lean thinking and the Productive Wards Programme are also attempts to improve the process of care. The responsibilities of nurses in management roles from ward sisters and team leaders through to directors of nursing, which involve planning, organising and co-ordinating care, are all essential functions to ensure safe, effective care that delivers good experiences for patients and staff.

Information box 2.1: Understanding quality improvement

Lean thinking: a methodology for looking at smarter ways of achieving outcomes and avoiding unnecessary waste. Originally developed by the Japanese company Toyota.

Productive Wards Programme: an approach used in the NHS to improving processes in a ward environment to facilitate nurses spending more time with patients.

One important difference between early theories of leadership which focused mainly on great leaders, and contemporary nursing leadership practice, is the expectation that all nurses as professionals are expected to lead, whether or not they have a management role. This includes you as a student nurse. Furthermore, modern thinking on leadership in healthcare specifically rejects the idea of heroic leadership, suggesting that leadership must be dispersed throughout the organisation. Turnbull (2011: 18) summarises this thinking very well:

> Leadership must be exercised across shifts 24/7 and reach to every individual: good practice can be destroyed by one person who fails to see themselves as able to exercise leadership, as required to promote organisational change, or who leaves something undone or unsaid because someone else is supposed to be in charge. The future of leadership and management in the NHS needs people to think of themselves as leaders not because they are personally exceptional, senior or inspirational to others, but because they can see what needs doing and can work with others to do it.

The most recent in a series of models developed to describe the nature of leadership in healthcare is the Healthcare Leadership Model (NHS Leadership Academy, 2013).

It is an attempt to define effective leadership in healthcare, and it recognises the importance of personal characteristics as did the early advocates of trait theory by stating that:

> The way that we manage ourselves is a central part of being an effective leader. It is vital to recognise that personal qualities like self-awareness, self-confidence, self-control, self-knowledge, personal reflection, resilience and determination are the foundation of how we behave. (NHS Leadership Academy, 2013: 3)

The model goes on to define the desired behaviours needed for effective leadership. The nine leadership behaviours identified within this model are listed in information box 2.2.

Information box 2.2: Nine leadership behaviours from the Healthcare Leadership Model

- Inspiring shared purpose.
- Leading with care.
- Evaluating information.
- Connecting our service.
- Sharing the vision.
- Engaging the team.
- Holding to account.
- Developing capability.
- Influencing for results.

As you can see, these behaviours are linked to the values of safe and effective care, and good relationships between the individuals providing care. Some behaviours in the model are dependent on the leader also having a management role. For example, the behaviour identified as 'developing capability' focuses mainly on providing opportunities for learning, something that may be facilitated with the support of managers for the member of staff. Building capability is also about the way in which opportunities for learning are facilitated and promoted for patients – when you come to read about 'collective leadership' in Chapter 9 you should be able to see how patients should be included in that collective. The dimension of 'inspiring shared purpose' speaks of acting as a role model for the values of the service, and having self-confidence to question the way things are done. It is important to point out that not all staff will display the full range of behaviours, with only very senior or experienced practitioners getting to that point. However, you as a student nurse should work towards the development of these behaviours – leadership development is a process and one that requires experience.

HEALTH ORGANISATIONS – COMPLEX SYSTEMS, COLLECTIVE LEADERSHIP

Knowing how organisations work is an important aspect for your development and impacts on your ability to give good care to patients. By knowing the priorities of the organisation, how decisions are made and where to go for guidance you can be more effective as a leader. In the same way that theory around leadership and management has evolved, so too have the management/leadership systems governing health organisations, moving from simple management structures with primarily consultant-led decision making supported by hospital administrators, to overarching governing boards with complex decision-making systems and processes. Historical reports have detailed the need to improve leadership and management to deliver good care using funding effectively and efficiently. A key report in 1983, the Griffiths report, resulted in the introduction of general managers, many of whom became chief executives in the 1990s. Nursing leadership was largely absent from this report. Thus clinical leadership became widely interpreted as medical. (That is not to say that nurses did not become chief executives or clinical directors.) *The NHS Plan* in 2000 (Department of Health, 2000) introduced the concept of performance and standards with annual assessments and published results. The most radical reform and most difficult to navigate was set out in *Liberating the NHS* in 2010 (Department of Health, 2010) and came into practice in 2012. To help people understand the most recent reforms, the NHS in May 2013 produced a *Guide to the Healthcare System in England* which explains how NHS-funded services are delivered in a wide range of organisations – NHS provider organisations include providers of primary and secondary care and other providers of health services such as charities, private organisations and social enterprises – and how collectively the organisations make up the healthcare system. In addition The King's Fund has produced an informative yet simple alternative guide to the NHS (www.kingsfund.org.uk/projects/nhs-65/alternative-guide-new-nhs-england).

For those of you who live and work in Scotland, Wales or Northern Ireland, the following links take you to information that tells you more about the NHS in those countries:

- For Scotland: www.show.scot.nhs.uk/organisations
- For Wales: www.wales.nhs.uk/governance-emanual/organisational-structure
- For Northern Ireland: http://online.hscni.net

DRIVERS FOR CHANGE

Chapter 3 highlights the complex and political nature of the NHS and the impact on organisations in which healthcare is delivered. It also sets out key drivers for change including the overwhelming demand on health services due to a wide range of reasons, including an increase in the aging population with complex and multiple illnesses, alongside a diminishing budget in an economic climate constantly under review.

Recently in England the NHS *Five Year Forward View* (NHS England, 2014) set out a vision for the NHS, its main theme being the development of new models of care. A clear driver of the strategy is the objective of ending the classic divide between family doctors and hospitals, and between physical and mental health, as well as between health and social care, and prevention and treatment. The Health Foundation (an independent charity working to improve the quality of healthcare in the UK) has recently suggested there is agreement that the main challenges for healthcare over the next five years are:

- Achieving financial balance.
- Transforming the way care is delivered for the future.
- Maintaining and improving the quality of care and health.

They also suggest that failing to meet any one of the above would have serious consequences for the NHS and the care patients receive. It is important to stay mindful of the overarching context and challenges to better understand the impact on the local organisations in which you are placed, and why these might give rise to variations in the quality of care and patient and staff experience.

Activity 2.2

- Pause for a moment and think about the many policy changes in the UK that are impacting on our healthcare organisations.
- What impact does this have on you as a student nurse? What impact will these changes potentially have on your approach to leadership; both positive and negative?

BOARD STRUCTURE AND RESPONSIBILITIES

NHS Boards across the UK are made up of executive and non-executive directors from a range of backgrounds including finance, clinical (medical and nursing director posts are mandated on an NHS Board), as well as lay members of the public who can apply to be non-executive members. Individuals are recruited according to organisational needs and the skills gaps identified amongst existing Board members. You may wish to access websites that tell you which Boards are in your UK country, and how these are governed (Scotland – www.gov.scot/Topics/Health/NHS-Workforce/

NHS-Boards; England – www.nhs.uk/NHSEngland/thenhs/about/Pages/nhsstructure .aspx; Northern Ireland – http://online.hscni.net/other-hsc-organisations; Wales – www.wales.nhs.uk/ourservices/directory/LocalHealthBoards).

The Board is responsible and accountable for vision, strategy and leadership, and for ensuring that the strands of NHS governance are in place to achieve high standards of patient care. Governance means taking responsibility for the processes and structures that guide an organisation, including risk management, clinical standards, finance controls, assurance, probity (decency, integrity) and ethics of the organisation. These are important concepts, probably not all of which will be familiar to you, and are explained in more detail in *The Nurse Executive's Handbook: Leading the Business of Caring from Ward to Board* (Burdett Trust for Nursing and the King's Fund, 2009) which you may find useful. The role of the Board is described on p. 16 of that publication and is reproduced in information box 2.3.

Information box 2.3: The Board's role

The role of the NHS Board is to:

- Be collectively responsible for adding value to the organisation, for promoting the success of the organisation by directing and supervising the organisation's affairs.
- Provide active leadership of the organisation within a framework of prudent and effective controls which enable risk to be assessed and managed.
- Set the organisation's strategic aims, ensure that the necessary financial and human resources are in place for the organisation to meet its objectives, and review management performance.
- Set the organisation's values and standards, and ensure that its obligations to patients, the local community and the Secretary of State are understood and met.

Find out more in *Governing the NHS: A Guide for NHS Boards* at: www.dh.gov.uk

---

The local NHS leadership within an organisation is not just directly responsible for the overall leadership strategy but also for how this gets communicated and lived out in the day-to-day running of organisations, with this varying significantly depending on the type and size of organisation (acute, community, mental health, etc.). The responsibility for the overall leadership of the organisation is an example of *collective leadership*. Collective leadership is a relatively recent development in leadership thinking and suggests that large organisations cannot be effectively led by a great leader, or even several great leaders: the organisation needs many people exerting leadership working together. Collective leadership is discussed in more detail in Chapter 9.

THE IMPACT OF REGULATORS ON THE LEADERSHIP AGENDA

Organisations are held to account by a wide range of regulators, i.e. bodies that have a governance role in protecting the public and patient safety by the regulation of their members. Recent years have seen increased regulatory scrutiny as quality of care has rightly risen up the agenda following some major and high profile failings in care, with a number of recommendations and reports into patient safety, including the Berwick Report (National Advisory Group on the Safety of Patients in England, 2013), the Keogh Mortality Review (2013) and the Vale of Leven report (MacLean, 2014) in Scotland.

The Care Quality Commission (CQC) in England has a major role in inspection, and in 2012 was given increased powers to regulate services to meet agreed standards of care. Measuring the quality of healthcare and thus benefits to patients is a complex process. There are multiple definitions of quality, although it is commonly defined as care that is clinically effective, safe and provides a positive experience for patients. Other definitions are broader, focusing on key areas such as:

- Safety.
- Effectiveness.
- Person-centredness.
- Being respectful and responsive to individuals' needs and values.
- Being timely, efficient and equitable.

However, the measures used to assess whether an organisation is 'good' are not necessarily consistent, are hotly debated and may be open to interpretation. Whatever measures the organisation is assessed by, there is no system that measures the whole. At best the measures assess structures and processes which support effectiveness, assuming that if those are robust, the organisation as a whole will be more likely to provide safe, effective and humane care. It is important for you to be aware of these drivers and to understand the need for NHS providers to meet additional standards such as minimum staffing numbers, or consultant-led seven day services. It starts to become clear that there is a need for additional investment and expenditure – a political point and one which we are sure you are aware of given the ongoing media attention that the NHS receives. The impact of these drivers may tip organisations into financial debt, triggering a cycle of cuts which then impact on service delivery.

Organisations defined by regulators as needing to improve in the delivery of quality care, often find it difficult to operate beyond crisis management, which may give rise to autocratic styles of leadership, with varying degrees of hierarchical, controlling, directional traits, and perhaps short on nurturing, developing or collaborative approaches. In addition, the thinking around successful organisational management and leadership sets out a very different style of collective leadership, which is not just about personal characteristics defined within the healthcare leadership model but is also focused on organisational relations, connectedness and interventions into the organisational system, as well as changing organisational practices and processes (Turnbull, 2011).

Activity 2.3

Drawing on your experience from a variety of clinical placements, what things do you see, hear and experience that give you confidence in the quality of the service?

DIRECTOR OF NURSING AS LEADER

The complexity of the health and social care systems outlined in this chapter has ensured an increasingly multifaceted role for the executive nurse. Portfolios of responsibilities are diverse and vary to suit the type, size and nature of organisations, and may include areas such as organisational development, commissioning, transformation, clinical governance, complaints, marketing, education and research. A vital aspect of the role of a Director of Nursing is to inform and advise the organisation's Executive Board about how their decisions may affect the quality and safety of patient care and the wider patient experience. This may not be as straightforward or easy as it could appear. Much will depend on the skills, competence and leadership of the nurse director and their ability to look at the issues within the context of the organisation as a whole. (See Chapter 10 for further insights into nurse leaders who have been interviewed for this book.)

In her work at the University of Leeds, Professor Beverly Altimo-Metcalfe has identified key components of leadership that are relevant to the NHS and the public sector as a whole including:

- Showing genuine concern for staff and patients.
- Being accessible.
- Encouraging change.
- Being entrepreneurial.
- Resolving complex problems.
- Networking.
- Achieving results.
- Focusing team effort.
- Supporting a developmental culture.
- Facilitating change sensitively. (Alimo-Metcalfe and Alban-Metcalfe, 2006)

You may find this list useful when considering the qualities that are needed as a nurse leader, and in particular as a leader in an executive role. You may be an aspiring

Director of Nursing – if so, you can start to consider how you can go about building up the particular executive skills and qualities that you will need as you progress through your career.

LEADERSHIP DEVELOPMENT: FROM BOARD TO WARD

We have emphasised the role of the Board in setting the leadership direction for a healthcare organisation – and to do this with clarity of strategic purpose – but little can be achieved if the Board fails to integrate good leadership principles across the organisational structures. These will vary, but generally below the Board Directors there are strategic leaders who head up business units – for example, surgery, medicine, women's and children's services, and emergency care. And of course, the structures in primary care are headed up by strategic leaders. The Divisional Directors are typically medically trained clinicians supported by general managers and matrons. The structures are often hierarchical with most commonly a medical lead, although the leadership may also be designed as a decision-making collaborative. Alongside the leadership roles are management responsibilities, including targets around delivery. Across the UK, the NHS has slightly different structures in place – for example, NHS Boards in Scotland compare to NHS Trusts in England yet will still have an Executive 'board' of leaders to lead the organisation in the services and quality of services they provide.

In addition, organisations often have government or local authority targets to achieve. These targets may be multiple and often complex to deliver – for example, infection and pressure ulcer rates, national waiting times, and the Friends and Family Tests are all important quality assurance measures of the way that care is delivered and require to be monitored and reported. Financial management is also complex and essential for ensuring the organisation is paid for the work it delivers and comes in within budget. These indicators, amongst others, are used to judge how effectively the organisation is led and managed. 'Metrics that matter' are those that facilitate good decision making based on good relevant information – an important concept as you navigate the data that are available in practice. The aim is to empower individuals to continually improve care within a climate of trust. Evidence is starting to show that collective leadership is a facilitator for the delivery of safe, effective care (e.g. Salford Royal as cited in King's Fund, 2014).

SUMMARY

Some key points from this chapter include:

- The systems in which you deliver care are multi-faceted and complex, and you have a responsibility to understand those complexities.

- Leadership and management skills, knowledge and attributes bring different things to different situations. Leaders need to be 'nimble' in their abilities to use different approaches.
- You can begin to develop your portfolio of leadership skills with an eye on your own career path.

FURTHER RESOURCES

The reading that we recommend are the websites that we have already mentioned – as a way for you to compare and contrast the NHS across the UK, and as a focus for you to stay up to date with the NHS in the country within which you work. They are as follows:

Scotland: www.gov.scot/Topics/Health/NHS-Workforce/NHS-Boards
England: www.nhs.uk/NHSEngland/thenhs/about/Pages/nhsstructure.aspx
Northern Ireland: http://online.hscni.net/other-hsc-organisations
Wales: www.wales.nhs.uk/ourservices/directory/LocalHealthBoards

To access further resources related to this chapter, please visit the companion website at https://study.sagepub.com/taylor

REFERENCES

Alimo-Metcalfe, B. and Alban-Metcalfe, J. (2006) 'More (good) leaders for the public sector'. *International Journal of Public Sector Management*, 19(4): 293–315.

Burdett Trust for Nursing and the King's Fund (2009) *The Nurse Executive's Handbook: Leading the Business of Caring from Ward to Board*. King's Fund London. [Online] Available at www.kingsfund.org.uk/projects/ward-board-nurse-leadership. Accessed 12/9/2016.

Carlyle, T. (1841) *On Heroes, Hero Worship and the Heroic in History*. London: James Fraser.

Covey, S. (1992) *Principle-centred Leadership*. London: Simon and Schuster.

Department of Health (2000) *The NHS Plan*. London: HMSO.

Department of Health (2010) *Equity and Excellence: Liberating the NHS*. London: HMSO.

Fiedler, F.E. (1967) *A Theory of Leadership Effectiveness*. New York: McGraw-Hill.

Griffiths, R. (chair) (1983) *NHS Management Inquiry*. London: HMSO. [Online] Available at www.sochealth.co.uk/national-health-service/griffiths-report-october-1983. Accessed 12/9/2016.

Hersey, P. and Blanchard, K. H. (1969) *Management of Organizational Behavior – Utilizing Human Resources*. New Jersey: Prentice Hall.

Keogh, B. (2013) Review into the Quality of Care and Treatment Provided by 14 Hospital Trusts in England: Overview Report. [Online] Available at www.nhs.uk/NHSEngland/bruce-keogh-review/Documents/outcomes/keogh-review-final-report.pdf. Accessed 12/9/2016.

King's Fund (2014) *Developing Collective Leadership for Health Care*. London: King's Fund.

King's Fund (2015) *Alternative Guide to the New NHS England*. [Online] Available at www.kingsfund.org.uk/projects/nhs-65/alternative-guide-new-nhs-england. Accessed 12/9/2016.

MacLean, R. (2014) *The Vale of Leven Hospital Inquiry Report*. Scottish Government: APS Group.

National Advisory Group on the Safety of Patients in England (2013) *A Promise to Learn – A Commitment to Act – Improving the Safety of Patients in England.* [Online] Available at www.gov.uk/government/uploads/system/uploads/attachment_data/file/226703/Berwick_Report.pdf. Accessed 12/9/2016.

NHS (2013) *Guide to the Healthcare System in England Including the Statement of NHS Accountability.* Available at www.gov.uk/government/uploads/system/uploads/attachment_data/file/194002/9421-2900878-TSO-NHS_Guide_to_Healthcare_WEB.PDF. Accessed 16/06/2016.

NHS England (2014) *Five Year Forward View.* [Online] Available at www.england.nhs.uk/wp-content/uploads/2014/10/5yfv-web.pdf. Accessed 12/9/2016.

NHS Leadership Academy (2013) *The Healthcare Leadership Model,* version 1.0. Leeds: NHS Leadership Academy.

Nursing and Midwifery Council (2010) *Standards for Pre-registration Nursing Education.* London: NMC.

Spencer, H. (1896) *The Study of Sociology.* London: Appleton.

Stanley, S. (2009) 'Clinical leadership and the theory of congruent leadership'. In: Bishop, V. (ed.), *Leadership for Nursing and Allied Health Care Professionals.* Berkshire: McGraw-Hill.

Stogdill, R.A. (1974) *Handbook of Leadership: A Survey of Theory and Research.* New York: Free Press.

Taylor, R. (2009) 'Leadership theories and the development of nurses in primary healthcare'. *Primary Health Care,* 19(9): 40–5.

Turnbull, J.K. (2011) *Leadership in Context: Lessons from New Leadership Theory and Current Practice.* [Online] Available at www.kingsfund.org.uk/sites/files/kf/Leadership-in-context-leadership-theory-current-leadership-development-practice-Kim-Turnbull-James-The-Kings-Fund-May-2011.pdf. Accessed 12/9/2016.

Weber, M. (1905) *The Protestant Ethic and the Spirit of Capitalism: And Other Writings.* New York: Penguin.

3 POLICY PERSPECTIVE

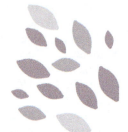

Students as the future generation of leaders

Lizzie Jelfs

Chapter learning outcomes

On completion of this chapter you will be able to:

- Define policy and explain the basic health policy-making structures across the UK.
- Identify some of the core assumptions and biases that have a particular impact on policy for nursing.
- Understand major current health policy trends that have a particular bearing on nursing and articulate some of the implications for future nursing leaders.
- Explain a range of core components for influencing policy and apply that knowledge through case studies of policy influencing.

Key concepts

Health policy, nursing policy, politics, influencing skills

INTRODUCTION

Be honest, did you see the title of this chapter and inwardly groan? Policy often conjures up negative images: dusty reports left forgotten on a shelf; committees full of people in suits who understand little of the realities of working in healthcare; a frustrating set of rules that stop you doing what you need to do but that you're powerless to change.

Part of my aim in this chapter is to persuade you that health policy is more interesting than you might think. But more importantly, I want to convince you that understanding and influencing policy is vital for all future nursing leaders: that having well-functioning 'policy antennae' will serve you well wherever you work. I want to do that by considering policy from four different angles. First, I'll spend some time pinning down what is meant by 'policy' and walk through the important structures in the UK for policy-making. Second, I'll explore assumptions and biases that shape policy on nursing. Third, I'll look at some of the important health policy trends that have a particular impact on nursing and consider their implications for you as a future leader. Lastly, I'll focus on important factors for influencing policy based on two case studies.

WHAT IS POLICY AND WHY DOES IT MATTER?

What is policy?

Let's start by looking at what is meant by the term 'policy'. *The Chambers Dictionary* defines policy as follows:

> Policy noun: 1. A plan of action, usually based on certain principles, decided on by a body or individual. 2. A principle or set of principles on which to base decisions. 3. A course of conduct to be followed. 4. Prudence; acumen; wisdom.

This is a helpful place to start. What you can see is that each of the four definitions captures a different facet of policy. The first and second definitions show that policy is usually based on principles; policy is about underlying ideas. But you can also see that policy isn't just about a theoretical discussion. As the first definition suggests, in policy there are principles that are meant to drive a plan of action. The third and fourth definitions also highlight something else that is particularly important for understanding policy: that it usually has a normative element. That is, it has a sense of setting standards and expectations, based on a judgement of what it supposes to be the right course of action. As you'll see, this aspect is important for understanding health policy, and policy on nursing in particular.

In essence, policy is a framework that governs action: enabling certain things to happen and constraining others; setting expectations, directions of travel and boundaries. But it's not neutral. It expresses dominant ideas and political objectives; what people think are the right things to do.

Sometimes it is the principles underpinning a policy that change. For example, over time our society has developed expectations that patients and families are involved in their own care. This fundamental principle now underpins many policy decisions (see for example Department of Health, 2012). Sometimes, even where a principle has stayed relatively constant, the judgement on how best to enact it changes. For example, the principle of non-maleficence (that is 'first, do no harm' (*primum non nocere*)) has existed in medicine for thousands of years. The Hippocratic Oath contains the phrase 'to abstain from doing harm' and the origin of the specific Latin phrase can be traced back through at least three centuries (Smith, 2013). However, ways of putting this principle into action have changed. For example, in the UK and many other Western countries there has been an increasing focus in the past 20 years on patient safety, with different policy initiatives that seek to enact this, from the World Health Organization's (nd) *Safety Checklists* to safe staffing levels.

Why does understanding policy matter?

In this section, I explore why policy matters (or should matter) to nurses. The Nursing and Midwifery Council (NMC) is a good starting point for this part of the discussion.

> All nurses must act as change agents and provide leadership through quality improvement and service development to enhance people's wellbeing and experiences of healthcare. (NMC, 2010: 5)

> You put the interests of people using or needing nursing or midwifery services first. You make their care and safety your main concern and make sure that their dignity is preserved and their needs are recognised, assessed and responded to. You make sure that those receiving care are treated with respect, that their rights are upheld and that any discriminatory attitudes and behaviours towards those receiving care are challenged. (NMC, 2015: 4)

Policy, particularly beyond the organisational level, can easily seem remote from the realities of working life. What opportunity is there for an individual staff nurse, who is struggling to find staff to fill the rotas, to change big decisions on the numbers of nurses in the health service?

I want to make two points here. First, understanding policy and being able to critically analyse its main trends will help you hugely in interpreting changes that you see around you and taking opportunities as a leader. Since policy trends usually develop over time, being able to analyse policy will help you to adapt your own practice, or challenge policy directions that are to the detriment of the people in your care, whether those are users of health and social care services or the staff whom you lead.

Second, if policy is defined as a framework that governs action, then understanding and influencing policy are important aspects of every nurse's role. To act as a change agent and improve quality and services as the NMC standards expect, will inevitably bring you up against policy in one form or another. As you have already seen, policies are constantly evolving as the context of practice, the needs of patients and service users, technology and expectations change. Given that health professionals are governed by codes of practice that explicitly uphold good standards of care, with the service user and patient at the centre, your insights and input are vital to policy.

You may concentrate on influencing and leading policy within a local organisation or a team but you might equally choose to influence policy at a regional or national level. Whatever your decision, finding a voice, making yourself heard and making a persuasive case are part of the job for all nursing leaders.

Activity 3.1

Consider the areas of policy, relating to your own practice, that are of particular interest to you. Reflect on those aspects that you'd like to influence.

POLICY STRUCTURES

Overview of UK and home nation policy structures

Describing health policy structures is a thankless task. Aside from the complexity of describing numerous interlocking bodies, structural change in the NHS has been a constant theme for most of its existence. Most recently, the 2012 Lansley reforms in England, which abolished a range of regional and national policy-making structures, were described by the Chief Executive of the NHS who implemented them as requiring 'such a big change management [sic], you could probably see it from space' (*Health Policy Insight*, 2010). By the time you are reading this, it is likely that some of the structures I describe here will have changed. An additional complexity is that health policy is a devolved matter; that is, it is largely the responsibility of the English, Scottish, Welsh and Northern Irish administrations of the UK. This means that many of the structures are either different in the four home nations or replicated fourfold, and there are relatively few policy structures that are truly UK-wide.

Ministers

Each of the UK home nations has a senior government minister who is responsible for health policy at a national level. In England, there is a Secretary of State for Health, who sits in the Cabinet. This post is currently supported by a Minister of State for Health, whose responsibilities include hospital care, NHS performance, the workforce, and patient safety. There are also three Parliamentary Under Secretaries of State (junior ministers): one for Public Health and Innovation; one for Health (who sits in the House of Lords); and one for Community Health and Care, with responsibilities including adult social care, community services and cancer care.

In Scotland, health is the responsibility of the Cabinet Secretary for Health and Sport. The Cabinet Secretary has two ministers working to them: the Minister for Public Health and Sport and Minister for Mental Health. In Wales, the Minister for Health and Social Services is a Cabinet post within the Welsh Government. The Minister is supported by a Deputy Minister for Health. In Northern Ireland, the Minister for Health, Social Services and Public Safety is responsible for health policy.

Departments of health

Working to the minister, each of the UK administrations has a government department with strategic oversight for health: in England the Department of Health (DH), in Scotland the Directorate of Health and Social Care, in Wales the Department of Health and Social Care, and in Northern Ireland the Department of Health, Social Services and Public Safety.

In England, the DH is also surrounded by arm's length bodies (ALBs) and other agencies, each with a particular remit for different areas of health service delivery. Most importantly, NHS England is responsible for national leadership of the NHS, oversees clinical commissioning groups, and commissions primary care and public health services. NHS England's annual budget was over £100 billion in 2015/16 (HM Treasury, 2015). Then there are ALBs that range from having responsibility for public health (Public Health England) or litigation claims (NHS Litigation Authority) to NHS education and training (Health Education England) and business support to the NHS (NHS Business Support Agency).

The devolved administrations also have other agencies associated with the departments of health, although their smaller size means that these are fewer in number. For example, in Scotland the lead NHS education agency, NHS Education for Scotland (NES), functions as a special health board, reporting to the Scottish Government.

Activity 3.2

Which of the UK countries are you based in? Take this opportunity to look on the relevant website to see the scope of policy that is 'out there'.

Chief Nursing Officers

Each of the four UK home nations has a Chief Nursing Officer (CNO) who leads the nursing and midwifery profession in their respective countries, providing expert professional advice to government. In Scotland, Wales and Northern Ireland the CNO is based within government, usually alongside other lead professionals. At the time of writing, however, the English CNO is located in NHS England rather than the DH (the Chief Medical Officer is based in the DH), a split which introduces additional complexity to nursing policy in England.

Royal College of Nursing (RCN)

The RCN is a UK-wide organisation that is both a professional body for nursing and a trade union. It was founded in 1916 as the College of Nursing, gained the title 'Royal' in 1939, and was registered as a trade union in 1976 (RCN, 2015). The RCN has offices in each of the UK home nations, as well as regional boards across England.

The RCN's joint role as professional body and trade union has not been without controversy. In recent years, there has been particular focus on whether the organisation can effectively fulfil both roles. Most significantly, the final report of the second Francis Inquiry into the Mid Staffordshire NHS Foundation Trust recommended that the RCN split its professional body and union functions (recommendation 201) (Francis, 2013a). So far, however, the RCN (2013: 8) has resisted calls to change its structures, stating that 'On our dual role, we believe that the elements are complementary to one another and make us a stronger organisation'.

Nursing and Midwifery Council (NMC)

The NMC is the professional regulator for both nursing and midwifery. The NMC's core purpose is public protection, through establishing and maintaining the register of nurses and midwives who can practise in the UK. Like most of the other eight health professional regulators, the NMC is one of the few UK-wide health organisations. The NMC is also the largest of all the UK regulators, with a register of more than 670,000 professionals. This compares, for example, with 270,000 doctors on the General Medical Council's register and 26,000 registrants with the General Optical Council. The scale and complexity of the register automatically make the NMC's work more challenging.

The NMC sets the Code (the standards for conduct, performance and ethics) for nurses and midwives and the standards for education that allow universities to provide programmes that lead on to professional registration. These standards include pre-registration education, standards for learning and assessment in practice and specialist qualifications (such as district nursing). From April 2016, the NMC is also responsible for a system of revalidation for all nurses and midwives, where registrants need to declare their continued fitness to practise every three years to remain on the register, based on a set number of hours of continued professional development (CPD) and reflection on feedback from colleagues, patients or others.

Set up in 2002 to take over the functions of the UK Central Council for Nursing, Midwifery and Health Visiting and the English National Board, which had particular responsibility for quality assurance of education, the NMC has had a number of critical reviews and changes of leadership over the past 13 years. Since an excoriating assessment by the Council for Healthcare Regulatory Excellence in 2012 (the regulator of the health professional regulators, now the Professional Standards Authority) the NMC has made significant progress, although the accountability hearings of the NMC before Parliament suggest that substantial challenges remain (House of Commons Health Committee, 2013).

European Union policy

One of the additional complexities of nursing policy is the role of the European Union (EU). A detailed survey of EU health policy would be a book in its own right and I only have space to touch on it briefly here. Suffice to say that EU policy has historically acted as another framework that sits beyond local, national and UK policy, although the impact of the 'leave' vote in the UK's referendum on membership of the EU in June 2016 may change that. The reason why it is particularly important for nursing is because of the bearing it has on the ability of professionals to work in other EU countries. Adult nursing, also known as general care nursing, is one of the seven so-called 'sectoral professions'. This means that if you are a registered adult nurse or a midwife in the UK you have the right to be accepted onto the register of any other EU country, without additional requirements (known as compensation measures) and vice-versa.

As a consequence, EU legislation sets out in some detail what it means to be a 'general care' nurse in legislation known as the Professional Qualifications Directive (2013/55/EU). A Directive is binding law so all EU member states have to follow it. It is written into our home legislation in the UK through a process called transposition. Directive 55 also sets the expectations on education, including an Annexe that lists the minimum content of education programmes. It is this legislation that is actually responsible for the amount of time you spend on your course, including the amount of time you spend in practice. Influencing the policy debate in Brussels is beyond the scope of this chapter but there are concerns that UK nurses and midwives could do more to strengthen their policy voice. A recent paper for the *Journal of Research Nursing* on the nursing policy context concluded that 'there is an absent voice at EU level from the European universities that contain nursing departments' and that 'there are continual threats to the integrity of nurse training and education – political and policy vigilance is necessary' (Gobbi, 2014). At the moment it is not possible to predict the impact of the referendum result on healthcare in the UK, but it is likely to take a number of years to negotiate the changes that would affect the automatic recognition of healthcare staff moving to work in the UK from other EU member states, and vice versa.

MUTATIONS IN THE POLICY DNA: UNDERSTANDING POLICY BIAS

Policy bias

So far, you might have the impression that policy is based on structure, process and legal frameworks. But as I flagged at the start of this chapter, policy is not just a rational 'plan of action' based on an objective assessment of worthy principles; it is also based on beliefs and a judgement on what is right to do – in other words, people's values and assumptions.

In the case of nursing, deeply ingrained assumptions about the profession create what one commentator has called 'a genetic mutation' in the policy DNA ('Grumbling Appendix', 2014). This means that there are certain ways of thinking that crop up time and time again in different policy debates on nursing. To use another analogy, it's like having a car that steers to the left: if you want to drive straight you have to constantly adjust for the bias. Keep looking for these ways of thinking as you analyse policy and you will find many more, but to get us started, here are two that have been important in the UK (although to different degrees in the different home nations) in recent years.

Care versus intellect

As a nursing student, you will doubtless already have come across the juxtaposition of the ability and willingness to care for people and intellectual capacity, particularly to complete a degree-level course of study. This argument crops up in various different forms: 'too posh to wash' (i.e. if a person has a degree they think that washing a patient or meeting other fundamental needs is beneath them) or 'too clever to care'. It is also associated with an assumption that degree-level education is delivered in 'classrooms', with nursing students not gaining any practical experience of 'hands on' nursing.

Bearing in mind that no student was implicated in the poor care at the Mid Staffordshire NHS Foundation Trust, the following quote from the Report of the Public Inquiry (Francis, 2013b: 1513) is interesting:

> The experience from Stafford, echoed by what emerged at the Inquiry seminars suggests that the current university-based model of training does not focus enough on the impact of culture and caring ... There should be an increased focus in nurse training, education and professional development on the practical requirements of delivering compassionate care in addition to the theory.

Although the cruder examples of this thinking tend to manifest themselves in the media, politicians also often fall into this way of thinking. Responding to the Francis Inquiry, the government (Department of Health, 2013: 19) foregrounded student nurses and a proposal that:

> Starting with pilots, every student who seeks NHS funding for nursing degrees should first serve up to a year as a healthcare assistant, to promote frontline caring experience and values, as well as academic strength.

Notice the assumptions: that nursing students don't already have prior care experience; that nursing students without that experience will have the 'wrong' values; that recruitment for nursing courses is based solely on 'academic strength'.

Activity 3.3

Consider what you have read so far in this section, and perhaps what you have seen in the media. Based on your knowledge and experience as a student nurse, what are your views about these assumptions?

One of the notable things about this mutation is that it does not affect other health professions. You will rarely hear a physiotherapist's or a doctor's degree-level qualification linked to a lack of ability to look after people (in fact probably the reverse). It is also a 'mutation' that differs across the home nations. In the context of the same education standards set by the NMC across the UK, you will hear the argument against degree-level nursing far less frequently in Scotland, Wales and Northern Ireland: this is a bias with a particular hold in England.

The essential logic that substantial problems in care now can be linked to degree level education is flawed at its very foundation. Although nursing degrees have been around as qualifications since the 1960s, graduates were in relatively small numbers until more recently. In a study of hospitals in nine European countries, England (figures aren't available for the UK) had the second lowest rates of graduate nurses within the registered nursing population that was sampled, with 28% educated to degree level (and levels that ranged from 10% to 49% between different hospitals). This compares to 58% in Ireland, 50% in Finland and 100% in Spain and Norway (Aiken et al., 2014). The logic is also undermined by the research evidence on mortality. In the same study, it was found that a 10% increase in the proportion of nurses holding a bachelor's degree was associated with a 7% decrease in the risk of death after surgery.

Putting logic aside, if you want to understand and influence policy you have to get to grips with and learn how to refute the bias that for a nurse, a high level of knowledge, critical thinking and research awareness are somehow associated in some people's minds with deficient rather than high quality care.

Task orientation

Nursing as a profession is often portrayed in policy through the lens of a set of tasks of direct patient care: making sure that a patient's pain is managed; checking that patients are hydrated; completing care plans. Many of the inquiries that look at poor nursing practice focus on the absence of particular tasks being completed.

Although tasks such as these fundamentals of care are a crucial part of a registered nurse's role, it is problematic if nursing is seen exclusively through this lens. In particular, it underplays the role and responsibilities of the nurse as a health professional: making constant judgements in a range of complex situations, often working autonomously or leading teams of staff and moving between direct patient care and wider organisational work.

Davina Allen's (2014: 93) important research explores nurses' organising work: bringing order to patient care as nurses help patients navigate organisational boundaries based on 'a professional vision capable of zooming in and out from the individual to the many'. These complexities cannot be reduced to simple tasks, but without them the picture of nursing is incomplete. Allen concludes:

> There is a widely held view that all systems tend towards disorder and that energy is required to maintain order. Nurses are the source of this energy in healthcare. Formal organisations have a tendency to overestimate their orderliness and the degree to

which their activities are governed by rational systems and processes. Yet in so far as healthcare exhibits any order, the findings of this study show, this must be understood as a nursing order. (Allen, 2014: 150)

The second disadvantage of a task-focused approach to nursing is that the tasks that come under the spotlight are also often directed towards those surrounding the care of patients in hospitals. This tends to precipitate a focus on hospital settings, when in fact a large proportion of the NMC's register is working outside NHS settings and outside hospitals. It also risks confusion between the role of registered nurses and those who are working as care assistants or support workers. As support workers, particularly those working in higher level support roles, can be carrying out tasks that might be also completed by a registered nurse, a task-focused view of nursing fails to capture the unique value and contribution of the role of nurses.

Again, this is a bias that is particularly problematic for nursing. Although this approach can be seen to an extent with doctors (for example in the concept of 'task-shifting' to other professions and in some of the description of the emergence of new roles such as physicians' assistants), the strong and relatively cohesive medical professional identity means that it is both less prevalent and less problematic. We'll come back to this particular policy mutation later in the chapter in the case study on influencing the revision of the NMC Code.

THE HEALTH AND SOCIAL CARE MODERNISATION AGENDA AND ITS IMPLICATIONS

A core argument of this chapter is that being able to analyse and interpret policy trends is a vital part of your leadership role. This section briefly introduces a number of emerging policy trends and considers some of the potential implications for you as a future nursing leader.

Integration

Politicians in each of the UK home nations are committed to integration, although this is often ill-defined. Integration is usually shorthand for the bringing together either of health and social care (sometimes called horizontal integration) or hospital and community or primary care (sometimes called vertical integration). There are many different ways of understanding and implementing integration, from legislation to budget pooling. Nor is this a new trend; there have been numerous attempts over 30 years to bring services together in a way that makes the service user experience more seamless, including long-standing structural integration in Northern Ireland and more recent legislation in Scotland.

Although there is a particular impetus, not least economic, behind the current push for integration, the realities of implementing genuinely seamless services are far more challenging (Glasby and Dickinson, 2014). Finding ways to articulate and challenge the gap between policy rhetoric and practical reality for health professionals and service users is therefore a particularly important role for future nursing leaders.

Co-production with service users and carers

One of the most striking shifts in the provision of health and social care services in the past 40 years has been the changing relationships between health professionals and those who use services. This change is the subject of a substantial literature in its own right, which is worth further investigation. In essence, as society and patterns of disease have changed, those who use health and social care services increasingly expect to be involved in their own care rather than passive recipients, particularly if their condition is long-term and chronic.

Policy documents across all four UK home nations have increasingly reflected this aspiration for 'co-production'. This aspiration ranges from the Department of Health in England's 2012 consultation *Liberating the NHS: No Decision about Me without Me*, to the ambition in Scotland's *Quality Strategy*, for 'mutually beneficial partnerships between patients, their families and those delivering healthcare services' (Scottish Government, 2010). It has also been reflected in the NMC's 2010 nursing pre-registration education standards, which introduced an explicit expectation of service user involvement, something that is now routine in many parts of the curriculum across pre-registration programmes (see Chapter 5).

Enacting co-production requires a significant shift of mindset and new ways of working. As a future nursing leader, this ongoing shift will have a profound impact on your professional role, both in relation to service users and in relation to leading staff teams.

Multi-professionalism and the team

The relationship between professions and the way in which teams work together is an important policy trend. It has strong links to co-production, since patients experience health and social care primarily from a team, and it also has strong links to quality and safety, since there is good evidence that quality and safety of care strongly relate to how teams function. The 2015 Report of the Morecambe Bay Investigation, for example, highlighted the 'extremely poor' relationships between midwives, paediatricians and obstetricians as a key factor in the 'lethal mix' that resulted in 11 babies and one mother dying unnecessarily (Kirkup, 2015).

Although you will be familiar with inter-professional learning and team working from your pre-registration course, as integration is pursued the ties between professions and the additional complexities of team working beyond traditional health and social care professional relationships (for example, with police or fire officers) are likely to become increasingly important.

Another area in which the team may become more important in future years is that of regulation. As things currently stand, regulation is broadly divided into 'system' regulators, such as the Care Quality Commission (CQC), which looks at the organisation as a whole, and the professional regulators, which are focused on the individual. In practice, since care is experienced and delivered in teams, there is a case to be made that the lack of a concept of regulation of teams is a significant missing link. This isn't to suggest that professional or system regulation will be superseded but we could reasonably expect more discussion about the role of teams and regulation.

Prevention of ill health

Another policy area that has waxed and waned over the years is the prevention of ill health and promotion of health and wellbeing, also known as public health. Although there have been multiple policy documents setting out the aspiration to move from 'illness' to 'wellness' models, in order to improve the overall health of the population and reduce pressure on health services, actual improvements in public health have often proved difficult to achieve.

In Scotland, the *2020 Vision* for health states its aspiration for 'a healthcare system where we have integrated health and social care, a focus on prevention, anticipation and supported self-management' (Scottish Government, 2011: 1).

In England, the *Five Year Forward View* is, at the time of writing, the latest key policy document to set out the aspiration to foreground public health. Its challenge on public health is front and centre:

> If the nation fails to get serious about prevention then recent progress in healthy life expectancies will stall, health inequalities will widen, and our ability to fund beneficial new treatments will be crowded-out by the need to spend billions of pounds on wholly avoidable illness. (NHS England, 2014: 7)

Given the well-described and significant public health challenges for most Western nations, understanding your role as a wider public health practitioner, whatever your setting, is likely to become increasingly important as a nursing leader.

Activity 3.4

You might like to access the *Five Year Forward View* – for whichever of the UK countries (or elsewhere) you are based in – and use it as a basis to consider your role as a wider public health practitioner. Jot down your key points for further reflection as you continue to analyse your own leadership role.

INFLUENCING POLICY

Unfortunately there is no blueprint for influencing policy, or at least not one that I've discovered. Due to the inherent complexity of the way that policy is developed and shaped, it can be difficult to know which ideas will gain support and which will be dismissed. Evidence, as you'll see, is sometimes listened to but is frequently ignored; even influential individuals in positions of power sometimes struggle to persuade decision-makers. This should not, however, put you off seeking to influence policy. The final section of this chapter focuses on two case studies about influencing policy at a national level and some practical tips for getting into a policy debate.

Case study 3.1: Safe Staffing Alliance

For a number of years prior to the founding of the Safe Staffing Alliance there had been concern that nurse staffing levels were dropping. In 2012, the RCN published a document entitled *Overstretched. Under-resourced* (Buchan and Seccombe, 2012), highlighting the pressures on the workforce and concluding that:

> Workforce scenarios in NHS England strongly point to the likelihood of reduced supply of NHS nurses over the next five to 10 years. (Buchan and Seccombe, 2012: 1).

In 2012 both the RCN and the Council of Deans of Health UK had warned that cuts in the numbers of nurse education places were storing up future trouble in the domestic supply of registered nurses. These reports and calls had little effect on national policy, in part due to the call for the NHS in England to make £20bn in 'efficiency savings', which was dominating the agenda, particularly through the Quality, Innovation Productivity and Prevention (QIPP) programme. For a summary of QIPP see http://ukpolicymatters.thelancet.com/qipp-programme-quality-innovation-productivity-and-prevention.

In January 2013 a group made up largely of senior nurses formed the Safe Staffing Alliance (SSA), 'to take a stand on staffing levels' (Snell, 2013: 12). The Alliance set out five 'New Year's Wishes' around the core aim of securing increased recognition of the importance of staffing levels for quality of care and patient safety:

- Minimum registered nurse staffing levels.
- Information for patients on registered nurse numbers.
- An annual review of nurse staffing.
- More power for clinical nurse leaders.
- New research on registered nurse staffing.

Although the Alliance's message of 'never more than eight' (that is, that it is unsafe for nurses to have more than eight patients each to look after in general care settings in the daytime) was relatively simple, the Alliance also made a point of basing its messages on research studies, compiling and distilling the available evidence.

Later that year, nursing was firmly in the spotlight in the wake of the publication of the second Francis Inquiry into the Mid Staffordshire NHS Foundation Trust, with findings that included a ratio of 40:60 registered nurses to care assistants. A focus on staffing levels, however, was not a given: although the Francis Inquiry did recommend that independent work was carried out on safe nurse staffing, the political focus was more on 'culture' in general, regulatory failings and the individual culpability of staff (particularly nurses).

As the SSA campaign continued, nurse staffing levels began to rise up the political agenda. In Wales, legislation is in progress to make staffing levels a legal requirement. In England, the National Institute for Health and Care Excellence (NICE) was tasked with reviewing the evidence for safe staffing levels and published its first guidance, for safe nurse staffing in adult inpatient wards in acute hospitals in July 2014 (NICE, 2014). The Secretary of State also mandated in November 2013 that monthly nurse staffing ratios should be made available to patients and families on a ward-by-ward basis. Although the practical reality of staffing and funding increasing nurse numbers is far from resolved and NHS England halted NICE's programme on safe staffing in June 2015, the SSA has put this topic at the centre of discussion.

The Safe Staffing Alliance highlights a number of lessons in influencing policy. The Alliance benefited from a clear message, presented in a way that politicians and members of the public could understand; it used research and evidence to support and illuminate its case; and it managed to harness the support of both individual leaders and organisations. Although the research evidence has sometimes been simplified in ways with which the SSA might disagree, the Alliance has challenged and changed assumptions about the priority of nurse staffing in a way that will have an impact on political discourse for years to come.

Case study 3.2: Influencing the NMC's revised Code

The revision of the NMC's Code: *Standards of Conduct, Performance and Ethics,* which came into effect on 31 March 2015, was carried out as part of the NMC's regular cycle of document review. It is important to note that this occurred in the context of three important national reports that the NMC explicitly acknowledged would affect the revised Code: the second Francis Inquiry's final report; Camilla Cavendish's review of healthcare support workers; and the report led by Baroness Neuberger into the Liverpool Care Pathway (NMC, 2014: 3).

The Code is fundamental to nursing and midwifery practice. As you will know, it is the document which governs the conduct of all registrants, against which registrants will revalidate, and is the overarching framework in which the standards for education sit. Work began in 2013 with an initial gap analysis; this was followed by two phases of public consultation (which ran until summer 2014). In December 2014 the revised Code was approved by the NMC Council, for launch in 2015.

The most important part of the consultation was the second phase, which presented the draft revised Code for comment through a series of consultation questions devised by Ipsos MORI (supplemented by a range of focus groups). Ostensibly, the response was positive: the evidence report on the consultation process recorded that:

> The proportion of individual respondents indicating that the language and tone of the document was 'good' and that the document was easy to read and understand was consistently greater than 80 per cent. (NMC, 2014: 7)

However, a range of organisations had deep reservations about the draft. Aside from problems of duplication and a lack of clarity, these included concerns that the Code had become task-focused and dominated by the requirements of hospitals, rather than developing professionals with the judgement to take complex decisions across a wide range of settings. The RCN (2014) commented that:

> The RCN has significant concerns that despite best intentions, the NMC's work to develop the new model of revalidation and associated Code, has been too heavily influenced by recent public and political discourse. In seeking to address all recent and any future criticism of nursing and its professional regulation, the current draft Code lacks cohesion, clear purpose and strong, authoritative identity. (RCN, 2014: 1)

The Professional Standards Authority (2014), which regulates the health professional regulators, said:

> In our view, this draft is too prescriptive. The risk inherent in providing such a detailed set of standards is that gaps are likely to become apparent over time, and they will therefore require constant updating. A code based on more high-level statements can more easily address all the relevant areas, and is more resilient to future changes in policy focus. In addition, a very prescriptive set of statements leaves little room for a nurse or midwife to exercise professional judgement, thereby reducing the opportunities for professionalism to thrive. (Professional Standards Authority, 2014: 2)

Senior nursing figures from the UK home nations also wrote privately to the NMC. In response, the NMC revisited its draft and extensively redrafted its contents: unusually, the final draft of the Code that was approved by NMC Council was significantly different from the consultation version in May 2014.

This example sets out a different way of influencing policy. Here, existing consultation processes set in place by the NMC were used effectively by a range of organisations with similar concerns to reshape the policy outcome. Individuals (such as senior nurses) did play an important role but this was primarily the work of organisations, highlighting similar concerns even though they were not working together in any formal alliance.

OVER TO YOU ... SOME TIPS ON SHAPING POLICY

- Find your voice:

  An obvious point perhaps, but the first step is to be clear about what you want to say. There is no shortcut to this; it takes time to develop your knowledge and to understand the debates that you want to influence. There's no substitute for practice to enable you to know how to communicate what you think. When you do know your own views, spend some time thinking about how to put these across to others in a way that is clear and concise, particularly to those who aren't health professionals.

- Work out your best communication channels:

  Once you have a core message or a set of opinions there is a range of communication channels. Think about social media or print media; use opportunities to go to meetings where you can put forward your views; join committees and get involved with policy discussions.

- Understand and use evidence:

  As you've seen in the case study of the Safe Staffing Alliance, knowing and using the evidence to form your own opinions and then make your case is crucial. If you want your view to have weight, you need to know whether it has evidence to back it up and to be prepared to change your mind if the evidence isn't there.

- Develop relationships (alliances and individuals):

  Policy is usually developed by groups in discussion, both through formal routes of alliances and committees and through individuals. If you have an area of policy with which you particularly want to get involved, make contact with the key organisations and individuals that are active; over time, as you engage in discussion you will become more expert and your voice is more likely to be heard (see Chapter 8).

- Timing:

  Good evidence, clear opinions and an evidence-based argument can all fall flat if the timing isn't right. Keep an eye on the trends in policy debate and publication of key reports and inquiries, so that you can marshal your input at the right moment. Above all, be prepared to persevere. If your arguments aren't heard, their moment might not yet have come.

Activity 3.5

Are there organisations or committees that you could usefully become involved in? Find out more about these, and then make contact if you feel it is appropriate. (You might like to read Chapter 8 on 'networking' for some tips which aim to help you expand your networks.)

SUMMARY

The main aim of this chapter has been to make the link between your role as a future leader in nursing and understanding, interpreting and influencing policy. You have considered both the definitions and structures that underpin policy and the practical reality of policy in action: the biases that sometimes undermine nursing, significant trends in policy over the past few years and how you might start to influence policy.

Three key points to take away:

- Policy on nursing at a national level, particularly in England, is strongly affected by the history of nursing as a profession, which gives it 'mutations in the DNA': myths and biases that pop up in many different policy discussions. Understanding these and being able to shape, change and challenge them is an essential part of leadership.
- Policy is constantly evolving but there are key trends that you need to be aware of: in this chapter I have focused on integration, co-production, multi-professionalism and prevention of ill-health.
- Being able to influence policy is a combination of many factors. It is essential for you to find your voice and then the channels to communicate, basing your arguments on research and persevering until you've made your case.

FURTHER RESOURCES

These websites take you to the four UK country government websites for health. (If you are using this book outside of the UK, you will have your own country's website which you can access.)

Scotland: www.gov.scot/Topics/Health/About/Structure

England: www.gov.uk/government/organisations/department-of-health

Wales: http://gov.wales/topics/health/?lang=en

Northern Ireland: www.health-ni.gov.uk/

To access further resources related to this chapter, please visit the companion website at https://study.sagepub.com/taylor

REFERENCES

Aiken, L. et al. (2014) 'Nurse staffing and education and hospital mortality in nine European countries: a retrospective observational study'. *The Lancet*, 383: 1824–30.

Allen, D. (2014) *The Invisible Work of Nurses: Hospitals, Organisation and Healthcare.* London: Routledge.

Buchan, J. and Seccombe, I. (2012) *Overstretched. Under-resourced. The UK Nursing Labour Market Review 2012.* London: RCN. [Online] Available at www.rcn.org.uk/professional-development/publications/pub-004332. Accessed 30/05/16.

Department of Health (2012) *Liberating the NHS: No Decision about Me, without Me.* [Online] Available at http://webarchive.nationalarchives.gov.uk/+/www.dh.gov.uk/en/consultations/liveconsultations/dh_134221. Accessed 14/07/15.

Department of Health (2013) *Patients First and Foremost: The Initial Government Response to the Report of the Mid Staffordshire NHS Foundation Trust Public Inquiry.* London: DoH.

Department of Health (2014) *Jeremy Hunt: Message to NHS Staff One Year on from Francis Report.* [Online] Available at www.gov.uk/government/speeches/jeremy-hunt-message-to-nhs-staff-one-year-on-from-francis-report. Accessed 14/07/15.

Francis, R. (2013a) *Report of the Mid Staffordshire NHS Foundation Trust Public Inquiry*, Executive Summary. London: TSO, p.106.

Francis, R. (2013b) *Report of the Mid Staffordshire NHS Foundation Trust Public Inquiry*, Vol. 3. [Online] Available at http://webarchive.nationalarchives.gov.uk/2015040708 4003/www.midstaffspublicinquiry.com/sites/default/files/report/Volume%203.pdf. Accessed 14/07/15.

Glasby, J. and Dickinson, H. (2014) *Partnership Working in Health and Social Care*. Bristol: Policy Press.

Gobbi, M. (2014) 'Nursing leadership in the European landscape: influence, reality and politics'. *Journal of Research Nursing*, 19(7–8): 636–46.

'Grumbling Appendix' blog (2014, 29 April) '(W(h)ither Compassion?'. [Online] Available at https://grumblingappendix.wordpress.com/2014/04/29/whither-compassion. Accessed 14/07/15.

Health Policy Insight (2010) Editor's blog Thursday, 18 November: 'NHS CE Sir David Nicholson's speech to the NHS Alliance Conference'. [Online] Available at www.healthpolicyinsight. com/?q=node/858. Accessed 14/07/15.

HM Treasury (2015) *Policy Paper: Summer Budget 2015*. [Online] Available at www.gov. uk/government/publications/summer-budget-2015/summer-budget-2015#contents. Accessed 14/07/15.

House of Commons Health Committee (2013) *Accountability Hearing with the Nursing and Midwifery Council*, Fifth Report of Session 2013–14. [Online] Available at www. publications.parliament.uk/pa/cm201314/cmselect/cmhealth/699/69902.htm. Accessed 14/07/15.

Kirkup, B. (2015) *Report of the Morecambe Bay Investigation*. London: TSO, p.7.

NHS England (2014) *Five Year Forward View*. [Online] Available at www.england.nhs.uk/ wp-content/uploads/2014/10/5yfv-web.pdf. Accessed 14/07/15.

National Institute for Health and Care Excellence (2014) *Safe Staffing for Nursing in Adult Inpatient Wards in Acute Hospitals*. [Online] Available at www.nice.org.uk/guidance/sg1. Accessed 14/07/15.

Nursing and Midwifery Council (2010) *Standards for Competence for Registered Nurses*. London: NMC.

Nursing and Midwifery Council (2014) *Code Evidence Report*. [Online] Available at www.nmc. org.uk/globalassets/sitedocuments/consultations/2014/code-evidence-report.pdf. Accessed 04/07/15.

Nursing and Midwifery Council (2015) *The Code: Professional Standards of Practice and Behaviour for Nurses and Midwives*. London: NMC.

Professional Standards Authority (2014). *Response to the Nursing and Midwifery Council Consultation on a Draft Revised Code and Proposed Approach to Revalidation*, p. 2. [Online] Available at www.professionalstandards.org.uk/docs/default-source/publications/ consultation-response/others-consultations/2014/nmc-revised-code-and-revalidation. pdf?sfvrsn=7. Accessed 30/05/16.

Royal College of Nursing (2013) *Mid Staffordshire NHS Foundation Trust, Public Inquiry Report, Response of the Royal College of Nursing*, p. 8. [Online] Available at www2.rcn.org.uk/__data/ assets/pdf_file/0004/530824/francis_response_full_FINAL.pdf. Accessed 30/05/16.

Royal College of Nursing (2014) *Royal College of Nursing Response to Nursing and Midwifery Council's Consultation on a Draft Revised Code and Our Proposed Approach to Revalidation*. [Online] Available at https://www2.rcn.org.uk/__data/assets/pdf_file/0008/588365/44_14_

RCN_response_NMC_a_draft_revised_code_and_our_proposed_approach_to_
revalidation.pdf. Accessed 30/05/16.

Royal College of Nursing (2015) *Royal College of Nursing: Our History*. [Online] Available at
www.rcn.org.uk/about-us/our-history. Accessed 30/05/16.

Scottish Government (2010) *The Healthcare Quality Strategy for NHS Scotland.*

Scottish Government (2011) *Achieving Sustainable Quality in Scotland's Healthcare: A '20:20'
Vision.*

Smith, C.M. (2013) 'Origin and uses of primum non nocere – above all, do no harm!'. *The
Journal of Clinical Pharmacology*, 45(4): 371–7. [Online] Available at http://onlinelibrary.
wiley.com/doi/10.1177/0091270004273680/abstract. Accessed 14/07/15.

Snell, J. (2013) 'A nursing alliance with a firm and simple message: numbers matter'. *Nursing
Standard*, 27(18): 12.

The Chambers Dictionary, 21st Century Edition. [Online] Available at www.chambers.co.uk.
Accessed 14/07/15.

World Health Organization (nd) *Patient Safety Checklists*. [Online] Available at www.who.int/
patientsafety/implementation/checklists/en. Accessed 14/07/15.

4 LEADERSHIP AND INTER-PROFESSIONAL PRACTICE

Tim Bryson

Chapter learning outcomes

On completion of this chapter you will be able to:

- Draw conclusions about those aspects of working across professional boundaries that are most effective.
- Understand some of the barriers to inter-professional working and how these can be addressed.
- Understand the role of the nurse as a leader within inter-professional teams and across organisational boundaries.

Key concepts

Inter-professional working, inter-agency working, team leadership

---

INTRODUCTION

The purpose of this chapter is to demonstrate the need for good inter-professional working practices across health, social care and other sectors, with the nurse being seen as pivotal to the team. In this chapter I use the term 'inter' as opposed to 'multi' – not only for consistency and to hopefully avoid confusion, but also because it sits better with my interpretation of the purpose of inter-professional working which is about holistic integrated service delivery (as opposed to teams or individuals from different sectors simply coming together to deliver 'their' part of a package of care or support). I describe the context of inter-professional and inter-agency working – referring to many of the policy drivers that are described elsewhere in the book. I then go on to discuss team working and skills of leadership for inter-professional practice.

In Chapter 1, you looked at some of the historical leaders of nursing and, linked to that, the way in which nursing was seen as subservient to medicine. There can be no doubt that healthcare delivery and organisation of services have changed considerably over the years. Whilst there may still be some way to go, nurses are now seen as pivotal in delivering on the leadership and quality improvement agenda. I believe that the leadership challenge for nurses is to grasp this opportunity, in whatever role they occupy, and to take forward their leadership role in the design, implementation and evaluation of high quality patient-centred care, and in the context of inter-professional practice.

In order to take on that challenge, the traditional notion of nurses leading teams of nurses is not sufficient. This chapter explores the issues for nurses leading across professions, and leading across agencies and organisational boundaries, and provides a guide to that new style of leadership practice. As you might imagine, the key aim of inter-professional working is the enhancement of care so that people's experiences of health and social care are seamless and of the highest standards (Taylor and Brannan, 2014). Information box 4.1 gives find some definitions which will help you to draw out the key issues for inter-professional working, and to discuss some of the skills for working in such teams.

Information box 4.1: Definitions

- Inter-professional working: A group of individuals from different professions or disciplines working and communicating together.
- Inter-professional healthcare teams: Teams from different healthcare professions or disciplines working together towards common goals to meet the needs of a patient population. Team members work according to their scope of practice, share information to support each other's work, and co-ordinate processes and interventions in the provision of services.
- Multi-professional working: In general, the terms inter-professional and multi-professional are used interchangeably. It could be said that 'inter' refers to working practices that are holistic in nature, with 'multi' simply indicating that a number of different disciplines are working together.
- Multi-agency teams: This term is generally used for teams and services that include staff from the NHS, local authority social services, and the voluntary sector. The aim is to combine expertise and skills so as to offer a co-ordinated package of support and care to patients and their families.
- Inter-agency working: As with inter-professional working, the assumption is that inter-agency working involves working practices that are holistic in nature, bringing together practitioners from different sectors and professions to provide support for patients in an integrated way.

THE CONTEXT OF INTER-PROFESSIONAL AND INTER-AGENCY WORKING

The NHS is rarely out of the media headlines. I am almost sure that if you went to the news reports today (whatever day you are reading this chapter) you would be likely to find at least one news story associated with the NHS. As I am writing this chapter, I would suggest that information and stories about A&E waiting times and other missed targets, or about quality concerns, are as ubiquitous as the weather reports. Healthcare in the UK is facing massive challenges and is changing rapidly. Some of the key leadership challenges for nurses are about maintaining and improving quality of care at a time of highly constrained finances. At the same time, public expectations are rising, innovations in medicines and healthcare technologies are burgeoning, and population growth is placing increasing pressure on services. It has become increasingly recognised that high quality health outcomes can only be achieved through health and social care services working together far more effectively.

Activity 4.1

Make a list of all the professions, disciplines, services and organisations that you have come across in your time in placement. These may include social care services, charities, other hospitals or community settings.

The purpose of that activity was a simple one: to help you see the breadth of services, the range of professionals, and the scope of input available to you when you are working with patients to help them navigate the systems for their health and social care. When you listed these, you might have started to wonder about how these all 'join up'. This is where some of the legislative approaches in the UK come in, as well as some of the thinking from leading experts, as you will see.

Scotland has been one of the leaders in the development of legislation for the integration of health and social care (www.gov.scot/Topics/Health/Policy/Adult-Health-SocialCare-Integration). As the website states (Scottish Government, 2015):

> At its heart, health and social care integration is about ensuring that those who use services get the right care and support whatever their needs, at any point in the care journey.

Whilst there are different options available to make this happen, what is fundamental to success is, amongst other things, the engagement of stakeholders (health and social care professionals, the third sector, service users, carer, and others). Implicit within this engagement approach is the need, therefore, for health and social care professionals to find different ways of working. In their document entitled *National Health and Wellbeing Outcomes* (Scottish Government, 2015), an example is given of a case where an integrated approach to care is provided. It is summarised in case study 4.1.

Case study 4.1: A summary of Graham's story

(Taken from *National Health and Wellbeing Outcomes: A Framework for Improving the Planning and Delivery of Health and Social Care Services* www.gov.scot/Resource/0047/00470219.pdf.)

Graham is 55 years old, lives with his long-term partner and used to work with a local youth organisation. He is a volunteer. Graham was diagnosed with bipolar disorder when he was a teenager and received good support that enabled him to go to college and get the job that he wanted. When he was 45 he was diagnosed with heart disease. Graham found it increasingly difficult to manage his mental health effectively, partly due to the effect of his new medication on his moods and due to the stress of his diagnosis. Soon after his diagnosis, Graham's GP suggested he book a double appointment so they could talk through his diagnosis and what kind of support might help. The GP also referred him to the practice nurse and a social worker specialising in mental health. The practice nurse helped him understand his heart condition and how he could manage it. She also signposted him to a local cardiac rehabilitation group and the Citizens Advice Bureau. Through the social worker, Graham was put in touch with a peer support worker who helped him develop a Wellness Recovery Action Plan. As a result of the support he has received, Graham has been able to stay in work for several years following his diagnosis, and when he decided to retire he continued to do voluntary work.

Thinking about Graham's experience, you can see that a number of professionals were engaged in his care – an integrated approach to helping him identify and deal with his needs. However, I would assert that the situation described here is a multi-professional/multi-agency approach – one where a number of people from different professions offered their skills and expertise based on referrals from the GP and then onwards. The challenge perhaps could be to determine how this care pathway could be transformed into an *inter-professional* collaborative integrated pathway, maybe even with nursing at the heart of its leadership. These are thoughts aiming to provoke your own thinking – there are no right and wrong answers but you could consider these issues as you work in your own placement areas and see how patients flow through and across our systems and organisations (sometimes in ways where we may question how much control or autonomy they themselves have).

Moving on from this, the King's Fund is prolific in its critique and commentary on the issue of integrated care, which is so important when looking at inter-professional and inter-agency working practices (www.kingsfund.org.uk/topics/integrated-care). One example is the report written by Ham and Alderwick (2015) (*Place-based Systems of Care: A Way Forward for the NHS in England*) which summarises some of the strategic issues, namely:

- The pressures in the NHS are immense, including the financial constraints and demands.
- Care models need to be developed that will deal with the changing demands on health and social care.
- The organisation of the NHS has undergone many changes and it could be said it is in a state of fragmentation such as has not been seen before.
- Clinical service integration, rather than organisational integration, has been shown to impact positively.

Ham and Alderwick advocate for a more collaborative place-based system of care in order to deliver what is needed by the populations that the providers serve. In other words, there needs to be more of a focus on the pooling of resources, an integrated approach to service delivery, and changes in how that service is led and managed. The aim, of course, is to improve the health and wellbeing of the population. Scotland has already put in place the legislation for integrated care but Ham and Alderwick suggest that it could be taken further through this place-based system approach.

You may wish to access the website and 'travel the world' of integrated care to understand more about the challenges that we are facing here in the UK and globally. The King's Fund integrated care map (www.kingsfund.org.uk/topics/integrated-care/integrated-care-map) takes you from Cumbria in the UK to Noortalje in Sweden via Hospital in the Home in Victoria, Australia. The key message that comes through these case studies is that the needs of the individual or the population should be the starting point, not the model of working. However, the argument for *collaborative* approaches to the development of integrated services stands – though the model around which collaboration sits may differ depending on the context.

A further report by the King's Fund (Naylor et al., 2015) *Acute Hospitals and Integrated Care* recommends that if we are to address the changing needs of our population and manage the financial challenges, then acute hospital leaders have to move away from a hospital-based or organisation-based approach and move towards leadership across the health and social care system, and in particular integration between hospitals and primary care and between different hospitals. The report recognises that the evidence-base for the success of integrated care is still developing, but gives five case study examples. For example, in one case study the High Risk Patient Programme delivered by Northumbria Healthcare NHS Foundation Trust and partners has been associated with a significant drop in avoidable admissions and emergency readmissions.

As I have said, these challenges are not unique to the UK. The challenge of reducing costs at the same time as improving health outcomes and quality is faced across the developed world. In the USA, the Institute of Healthcare improvement (IHI) has proposed the adoption of a programme called the Triple Aim (IHI, 2013) which calls for action on three dimensions:

- Improving the patient experience of care.
- Improving the health of populations.
- Reducing the per capita cost of healthcare.

The US Institute of Medicine (IoM, 2015: 3) has recognised the crucial role that nurses can play in contributing to positive change in a rapidly evolving healthcare landscape, and it also emphasises the importance of inter-professional collaboration:

No single profession, working alone, can meet the complex needs of patients and communities. Nurses should continue to develop skills and competencies in leadership and innovation, and collaborate with other professionals in health care delivery and health system redesign.

This style of system-spanning leadership, rather than leadership that is solely focused within an organisation, is associated with better patient outcomes, fewer adverse events and greater staff satisfaction (Garner, 2011) and seems to reflect the place-based leadership approach described earlier. Nurses will need to rise to these challenges, and are often well placed to lead integrated teams and act as system or network leaders. Nurses work in a wide variety of settings and contexts, and all nurses can exercise leadership, whatever their role (Hasmiller, 2010). This point is made throughout this book as a call to action for you as a nursing student who has a role to play in the leadership of practice currently. Remember, you will have opportunities to influence and enhance practice and care as you progress to your newly qualified role and on to recognised leadership roles, possibly within integrated or inter-professional teams.

Activity 4.2

Think about one of the clinical placements that you have undertaken. Go back to your list from activity 4.1 of the services, professionals and agencies that were involved in the delivery of care.

- What was your perception of the working relationships, the accessibility of the services outside of the placement environment, and the integration of the pathway of care for patients?
- What is your view of the approaches to the way in which this clinical placement operated at an inter-professional or inter-agency level? Your collected observations aim to help you begin to build a view of excellence in inter-professional practice.

I hope you can see the clear policy directive towards integrated care. Whilst partnership working has been a feature of care historically, the focus now is on collaborative care – suggesting a shift from disciplines/professions working in parallel to achieve goals, towards professions working *together* with mutual trust and respect so as to achieve mutual goals (which of course are determined in collaboration with the patient). The evidence-base for inter-professional working is developing and Mitchell et al. (2013) have said that it has been linked to reduced hospital days, admission and improved performance, amongst other things. The current policy direction will have an ever-growing impact on the way in which you as an individual practitioner will work and it must mean that inter-professional and inter-agency working will become more and more important in the NHS. This leads me on to some of the skills that are required in this context.

INTER-PROFESSIONAL TEAMS AND TEAM WORKING

It is likely that you will have seen that all healthcare teams involve a degree of inter-professional working. Positive evidence of the impact of models of inter-professional team working is growing, particularly for teams working with patients with chronic diseases and mental health problems (Nancarrow et al., 2012). Nancorrow et al.'s study found:

- There is a need to change the way health and social care teams work so that care can be better – leading to, for example, a reduction in unnecessary hospital admissions, and facilitating early discharge.
- Interdisciplinary (their choice of term) team working is a complex phenomenon that depends on a number of aspects – context, leadership, purpose and vision, skill mix, service configuration, career development opportunities.
- Partnership (collaborative) working needs to be 'fostered and cultivated' (p. 183) with engagement of all staff across professional groups.
- The headline characteristics of a good interdisciplinary team are: communication, individual characteristics, leadership and management, personal rewards, training and development opportunities, quality and outcomes of care, appropriate skill mix, appropriate processes and resources, team climate, respecting and understanding roles, and clarity of vision.
- In advanced or mature collaborative teams, the patient and family are included as key members of the team.

Whilst teams can be effective and supportive, this is not always automatically the case and becoming a high-performing team takes effort and commitment by both team leaders and team members, with all members of the team having important roles to fulfil. Borrill et al.'s (2001) extensive research on inter-professional teams and team leadership identified the following key findings:

- Teams that work well together are more effective and more innovative than those that don't.
- The clearer the team's objectives, the higher the level of participation in the team.
- The greater the emphasis on quality and innovation, the more likely the team will be delivering high quality healthcare.
- Nurses working in well-functioning teams were less likely to leave their organisation or their profession (in the course of the year of the study).
- Team membership appears to buffer individuals from the negative effects of organisational climate and conflict in NHS hospitals.
- When diverse groups of professionals are in the team and working well together, then alternative and competing perspectives are carefully discussed, leading to better quality care decisions.

- Teams need to meet and to have effective meetings in order to build up a shared understanding of the work, and appropriate care processes.
- Lack of clear leadership is associated with poor team working, lower levels of participation, and lower commitment to quality care.

Borrill et al. go on to say that they believe that clear leadership involves:

- Creating alignment amongst team members around shared objectives.
- Generating enthusiasm and confidence for the work.
- Helping people co-ordinate activities.
- Helping individuals and the team as a whole to develop capability, and to continuously improve.
- Supporting team members to appreciate each others' contributions, and learning how to confront and resolve differences constructively.
- Building relationships with external stakeholders and helping to resolve conflicts between the team and others.

You may be thinking, how do I know how well a team is functioning? One way that you could start to consider this in your own practice is by using the lists here as a basis for reflection.

Activity 4.3

Using the two lists from Borrill et al.'s research and that of Nancarrow et al. described in this section, think about one of your clinical placements and the team working that you witnessed (and were a part of).

- What worked well?
- What didn't work so well?
- What could have been done differently to improve team working?

Your responses may indicate that the team that you work(ed) with integrated well with the services that feed into the patient pathways in that context. You may have experienced excellent inter-professional discussions leading to collective decision-making for patient care. You may also have seen leadership that enabled collaborative working relationships where different opinions were valued as part of the decision-making process. You may have had a different experience. This activity simply aimed to highlight some of the aspects of inter-professional team working that you can now look out for when you are in a new clinical placement. Whatever your experience, I hope you can see that the need for inter-professional working practices has never been more important. As a student nurse you will be moving in and out of different teams in your placements. You have a role to play in nurturing and valuing others, understanding the vision of your workplace, focusing on the patient and understanding their pathway and all those involved in their care, ensuring that the patient is at the centre and working with the inter-professional team in positive ways.

LEADERSHIP OF PEOPLE AND ORGANISATIONS ACROSS PROFESSIONAL BOUNDARIES

The traditional view of leadership may be one of seeing the leader as a charismatic hero coming to the rescue of a failing service or failing organisation – and sometimes you do see this where a Chief Executive of an NHS Trust or Board leaves following problems, and a new Chief Executive is brought in to 'solve all the problems'. However, it could be said that the challenges facing the NHS require a very different sort of leadership in which that leadership is shared and distributed amongst a broad coalition of clinicians and managers unified by a common purpose. Inter-professional and inter-agency leadership puts population and patient health outcomes first, and seeks to engage staff and engage patients in delivering a shared vision for improved care. Think about how nurses fit into this vision for a different kind of leadership. With their key clinical roles and the fact that they are commonly closer to the patient experience than perhaps some other professionals, it seems obvious that nurses therefore have a significant contribution to make.

The King's Fund has stressed the importance of roles that act as 'boundary spanners' (West et al., 2014). Boundary spanners can be defined as roles that may not necessarily have the power of senior positions, but they are able to make connections and engage across traditional boundaries. A powerful quote from this document is that 'Every interaction by every leader at every level shapes the emerging culture of an organisation' (p. 4). Given that inter-professional and inter-agency working requires cross-organisational collaboration, you can maybe see how complex it can be to work in this new integrated world of health and social care. However, if you can act as a boundary spanner, *you* can make real differences to the culture of care, and the overall way in which care is managed and delivered.

Leading across health and social care systems means that leaders need to:

- Develop and communicate a shared vision built on shared values.
- Have effective negotiating and influencing skills.
- Be emotionally resilient.
- Understand how the system works.
- Have change management skills.

So, as a student nurse you could well be in a position where you can act as a 'boundary spanner' – as someone who works across an organisation (or across more than one organisation), you will develop contacts and knowledge that could be useful as you move across the organisational boundaries. It is interesting to consider here what each profession may or may not understand about each other, and about the organisations that they work in. One of the barriers to inter-professional working is that lack of understanding associated with the different professional backgrounds from which teams are made up. Effective inter-professional teams are dependent on teams working in ways that offer a unified approach to care, using the skills and knowledge of team members in ways that may well cross boundaries (for the professionals involved) (Taylor and Brannan, 2014).

Activity 4.4

A number of key points have been made about inter-professional team working. You may wish to build on this learning by doing a short literature search on the nurse's role in inter-professional team working – perhaps with a focus on a clinical area of particular interest to you.

Anyone who has worked in a team will be aware that challenge and conflict can occur. Katzenbach and Smith (1993) suggest that challenge is necessary to teams but can be experienced as threatening. In their view, the crucial task is for a team to develop a strong sense of purpose and identity that reaches beyond the sum of the individuals involved, and that the team purpose helps to act as a guide for resolving conflicts.

The approach to conflict resolution adopted by Patrick Lencioni (2005) recognises that teams have common problems in becoming cohesive, and therefore in achieving their desired results. He believes that there are five key dysfunctions for a team: inattention to results, avoidance of accountability, a lack of commitment, a fear of conflict and an absence of trust.

It is also important to recognise that team leaders, such as ward managers or community team leaders, have a role in managing staff performance as well as supporting trust and involvement. An investigation into ward manager leadership styles by the Hay Group (2012: 3) found that:

> Leaders who consistently use the affiliative style often become too interested in creating harmony. They avoid uncomfortable performance management issues that need to be dealt with.

Leadership in any context can be complex, and the management of staff has a huge part to play – with leaders sometimes having to deal with difficult issues or conflict so that the team as a whole can work effectively within a framework of values. Linked to this issue of managing staff performance are the ways in which people in leadership positions can work positively with teams to hopefully prevent low staff performance wherever possible. High-performing ward managers demonstrated the following behaviours:

- Being clear about what is expected.
- Setting clear and challenging but attainable goals.

- Giving feedback and performance support.
- Enforcing only those rules and policies that are necessary, and minimising bureaucracy.
- Fostering a collaborative environment.

These leadership attributes relate well to the earlier discussion in this chapter on effective inter-professional team working as well as the way in which a leader can help individuals within a team to achieve their potential. You might like to think about a time when a team leader has helped you to further develop your skills in a particular situation so that you felt you were growing as a professional. Remember too that the skills listed here are not just the remit of a person in a leadership position, but are also skills that you as a student nurse can foster and demonstrate in your work, including as you work with a range of other professionals.

Other barriers to team working can include poor communication, inadequate knowledge about roles and professional identities, a lack of understanding about team working, a mismatch between policies across organisational boundaries, conflict related to hierarchy, uncertainty about decision-making and accountabilities, professional-specific language, management structures, and a possible lack of willingness to work together. Activity 4.5 aims to help you identify areas for your own professional development so that you can contribute to inter-professional teams positively and effectively – building on your current knowledge and skills.

Activity 4.5

Having worked through this chapter, consider all of the learning so far.

- What knowledge and skills do you think you currently have for inter-professional working?
- What knowledge and skills do you think you need to develop for your role as a student nurse in this context?
- And if you are almost at the end of your course, what knowledge and skills do you need as you move into your role as a newly qualified nurse?

I hope that you will have identified many of the attributes that you certainly will have at this stage of your learning. Perhaps you have excellent interpersonal skills and have been able to use these in situations where you have linked with social care professionals or others. You may have decided that an area you want to develop in is an understanding of other professions' roles. Whatever your current situation, the identification of what you are good at and where you need development is a fantastic starting point. The further resources offer some pointers to assist you, and it is likely that the resources within other chapters in this book will also assist you. Inter-professional working is here to stay – as it should be. You have a huge role to play both now and as you move forward in your career.

SUMMARY

The key points in this chapter are:

- Effective inter-professional, integrated, collaborative working approaches are crucial to the need for enhanced patient care (for example, to prevent avoidable hospital admissions, and to facilitate early discharge).
- Inter-professional teams and inter-agency teams, like any other team, require effective team leadership, team development and team review. If this leadership work is undertaken, patient outcomes and quality of care improve.
- Challenge, conflict and diversity are to be expected in teams and are an integral part of team leadership, and therefore to be welcomed rather than avoided.

FURTHER RESOURCES

Taylor, R. and Brannan, J. (2014) 'Interprofessional practice'. In: Lishman, J., Yuill, C., Brannan, J. and Gibson, A. (eds), *Social Work: An Introduction*. London: Sage.
A useful chapter written by a nurse (one of the editors of this book) and a social worker which provides an overview of the context and impact of inter-professional practice.

As discussed, Scotland has led on the development of legislation for the integration of health and social care. This website is a good resource demonstrating how legislation is developed and subsequently enacted: www.gov.scot/Topics/Health/Policy/Adult-Health-SocialCare-Integration.

The King's Fund website has multiple resources on integrated health and social care. These are accessible, evidence-based and are updated regularly so that you can keep track of the current situation: www.kingsfund.org.uk/topics/integrated-care.

 To access further resources related to this chapter, please visit the companion website at https://study.sagepub.com/taylor

REFERENCES

Borrill, C., Carletta, J., Carter, A., Dawson, J., Garrod, S., Rees, A., Richards, A., Shapiro, D. and West M. (2001) *Team working and effectiveness in health care: findings from the Health Care Team Effectiveness Project*. Aston: Aston Centre for Health Service Organisation research, Aston University. Available at Sro.sussex.ac.uk/54072/1/Andreas_FINAL_ACCEPTED-VERSION.pdf. Accessed 30/05/16.

Garner, C. (2011) 'A future where all nurses are leaders'. American Sentinel blog, 26 January 2011. [Online] Available at www.americansentinel.edu/?v=B&utm_expid=1046463-38.oWYf99mtTZat-3JVNJSejw.2. Accessed 14/02/16.

Ham, C. and Alderwisk, H. (2015) *Place-based Systems of Care: A Way Forward for the NHS in England*. London: The King's Fund.

Hasmiller, S. (2010) 'Nursing's role in healthcare reform'. *American Nurse Today*, 5(9): 68–9.

Hay Group (2012) *Nurse Leadership: Being Nice Is Not Enough*. London: Hay Group.

IHI (2013) *The IHI Triple Aim Initiative*. [Online] Available at www.ihi.org/engage/initiatives/tripleaim/Pages/default.aspx. Accessed 14/02/16.

Institute of Medicine (2015) *Assessing Progress on the Institute of Medicine Report: The Future of Nursing*. [Online] Available at http://iom.nationalacademies.org/Reports/2015/Assessing-Progress-on-the-IOM-Report-The-Future-of-Nursing.aspx. Accessed 14/02/16.

Katzenbach, J.R. and Smith, D.K. (1993) *The Wisdom of Teams: Creating the High Performance Organisation*. Boston, MA: Harvard Business School Press.

Lencioni, P. (2005) *Overcoming the Five Dysfunctions of a Team: A Filed Guide for Leaders, Managers and Facilitators*. San Francisco, CA: Josey Bass.

Mitchell, G.J., Cross, N., Wilson, M., Biernacki, S., Wong, W., Adib, B. and Rush, D. (2013) 'Complexity and health coaching: synergies in nursing'. *Nursing Research and Practice Annual*, 2013 (Article ID 238620): 1–7.

Mitchell, R.J., Parker, V. and Giles, M. (2010) 'When do interprofessional teams succeed? Investigating the moderating roles of team and professional identity in interprofessional effectiveness'. *Human Relations*, 64(10): 1321–43.

Nancarrow, S., Enderby, P., Ariss, S., Smith, T., Booth, A., Campbell, M., Cantrell, A. and Parker, S. (2012) *The Impact of Enhancing the Effectiveness of Interdisciplinary Working (Executive Summary)*. National Institute for Health Research Service Delivery and Organisation Programme. [Online] Available at www.nets.nihr.ac.uk/__data/assets/pdf_file/0009/85095/ES-08-1819-214.pdf. Accessed 14/02/16.

Naylor, C., Alderwick, H. and Honeyman, M. (2015) *Acute Hospitals and Integrated Care*. London: King's Fund. [Online] Available at www.kingsfund.org.uk/sites/files/kf/field/field_publication_file/acute-hospitals-and-integrated-care-march-2015.pdf. Accessed 14/02/16.

Scottish Government (2015) *National Health and Wellbeing Outcomes: A Framework for Improving the Planning and Delivery of Health and Social Care Services*. [Online] Available at www.gov.scot/Resource/0047/00470219.pdf. Accessed 14/02/16.

Taylor, R. and Brannan, J. (2014) 'Interprofessional practice'. In: Lishman, J., Yuill, C., Brannan, J. and Gibson, A. (eds), *Social Work: An Introduction*. London: Sage.

West, M., Eckert, R., Steward, K., and Passmore, B. (2014) *Developing Collective Leadership for Healthcare*. London: King's Fund. [Online] Available at www.kingsfund.org.uk/sites/files/kf/field/field_publication_file/developing-collective-leadership-kingsfund-may14.pdf. Accessed 14/02/16.

5 LEADERSHIP FROM THE PERSPECTIVE OF THE PUBLIC

Stephen Tee

 Visit the companion website at https://study.sagepub.com/taylor to watch Stephen discussing his chapter and his experience of leadership.

Chapter learning outcomes

On completion of this chapter you will be able to:

- Understand the role of nursing leadership in relation to the service user.
- Appreciate the policy origins of patient and public involvement (PPI).
- Describe a range of methods that support PPI in nursing leadership and understand how you, as a student nurse, could implement these.
- Evaluate the evidence for PPI and its impact on outcomes.

Key concepts

Patient and public involvement, nurse leadership, power, culture, collaboration

---

INTRODUCTION

This chapter explores nursing leadership from the perspective of the service user – people of any age, gender, ethnicity, religion, and including the wider family, carers and members of the public. It examines patient and public involvement (PPI) in nursing care and how such involvement can impact positively on quality, safety and health outcomes as well as the influence it has on nursing leadership. The chapter does this through a definition and discussion of PPI's policy origins, analysis of the organisational dynamics that impact on PPI, and the consideration of strategies and techniques that can bring about a change in practice. It is important to note that terminology varies within the literature and in policy. For the purposes of this chapter, I will use the term 'Patient and Public Involvement' (rather than, for example, 'Patient and Public Engagement' or 'Service User Involvement').

The last two decades have seen a significant shift in expectations in the UK pertaining to levels of accountability of all public sector services to the people that use them. Whether in health, social care, education or welfare, the public (including those that use services) expect a greater say in how such services are designed and delivered. This policy shift stems from two key drivers: the need for greater 'democratisation' and transparency around how taxes are used; and an attempt to increase competition and choice to drive up service quality. As a consequence of such policies, PPI in the process of design, delivery and service evaluation is now considered a routine part of the public sector leader's role. Nurses must increasingly be aware of how they can ensure the patient and the public voice is at the heart of their decision-making.

The skills of leadership have been shown to be vital to PPI and this chapter also includes an examination of the serious consequences of leadership failure and how genuine PPI can act as an important sense-check/barometer for those with responsibility for service quality and safety. As a student nurse you will engage with patients and the public on a daily basis when you are in clinical practice. Some of the issues within this chapter may be familiar to you, but it is vital that you consider the way in which PPI is conceptualised so that you can develop your leadership skills to enhance service delivery.

WHAT IS PATIENT AND PUBLIC INVOLVEMENT?

Patient and public involvement in healthcare is the process by which health service providers, such as a Hospital Trust or NHS Board, work together with ordinary citizens and patients to address complex organisational goals, such as the delivery of person-centred care (Patient and Public Involvement Solutions, 2012). It contrasts with previous approaches to health policy and delivery, which were characterised by a 'top-down' approach to decision-making, where 'experts', such as doctors, nurses and administrators, determined the shape of service provision without asking service users.

The top-down approach is no longer seen as appropriate in a highly complex world, with multiple inter-dependent agencies involved in healthcare delivery and where solutions require collaboration with stakeholders (including patients and the public) to deliver services that are responsive to diverse needs. Vignette 5.1 illustrates these points.

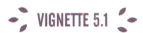

VIGNETTE 5.1

Professor Rosalynd Jowett is a member of the Board of Trustees for the Patients' Association (England). In that role she receives a great deal of feedback from people who use health services. She suggests that the NHS, even in 2015, still struggles with PPI, adding that the voice of the patient often remains unheard; that they are not seen as participants in their care and that their complaints are sometimes ignored. She argues that for nurse leaders to fully appreciate a patient's perspective, they need to step aside from their normal routines and think outside their day-to-day operational duties in order to see things from a patient's perspective.

Activity 5.1

List the key areas that make up patient and public involvement. Which of these have you seen taking place in practice? In your view, what are the areas that you as a student nurse can best contribute to?

Whilst robust research in the area of the impact or outcomes of PPI is somewhat limited and inconclusive, a number of Cochrane and literature reviews (Stringer et al., 2008; Wetsels et al., 2007; Lloyd, 2010; Tadd et al., 2011; Edwards et al., 2013) reveal evidence of:

- Improved patient satisfaction.
- Higher quality of care.
- Greater treatment compliance.
- Safer environments for patients and carers.
- Better health outcomes.
- Enhanced informed choice.

PATIENT AND PUBLIC INVOLVEMENT: A BRIEF POLICY OVERVIEW

In order to learn from PPI and facilitate your learning and development in this area, it is important to firstly understand some of the policy context (see Chapter 3 for the policy context). In the last decade or so, patient and public involvement has become an important focus of healthcare policy across the UK. *The NHS Plan* (Department of Health, 2000) outlined the shaping of services around the needs and preferences of individual patients. This was followed in 2007 by 'world class commissioning', which sought to embed PPI in the commissioning of services. *The Next Stage Review* (Department of Health, 2008) suggested that the NHS must seek to provide better information to patients and provide greater opportunity for participation, and that this must become a key measure of success. A significant step forward in 2009 was the publication of *The NHS Constitution* (Department of Health, 2009; NHS Choices, 2014a) which enshrined some important rights for service users – in particular the right of patients to influence their own care and local services. It states that as a patient or a member of the public:

> You have the right to be involved, directly or through representatives, in the planning of healthcare services commissioned by NHS bodies, the development and consideration of proposals for changes in the way those services are provided, and in decisions to be made affecting the operation of those services.

Each of the other three UK nations has identified 'constitutional' rights for service users (NHS Wales, 2015; NHS Northern Ireland, 2011; The Patient Rights (Scotland)

Bill, Scottish Government, 2011). You may wish to access the relevant document for the country that you are studying in.

In 2010 the UK coalition government's health White Paper *Equity and Excellence: Liberating the NHS* (Department of Health, 2010: 13) indicated that the chief goal of world-class healthcare:

> can only be realised by involving patients fully in their own care, with decisions made in partnership with clinicians, rather than by clinicians alone.

Liberating the NHS aimed to shift power from the centre (institutions) to GPs and patients (locally) and called for shared decision-making to become normal practice.

Of course shared decision-making can only become a reality where patients and the public have access to information on which to base their decisions and so the NHS has established the *Choices Framework* to support such a process. NHS Choices (2014b) provides a huge amount of information on services, conditions, treatments and research that aims to empower people. Similar policy initiatives exist in Scotland, Wales and Northern Ireland, and broadly sit under the banner of PPI, collectively seeking to empower people, giving control and choice.

The aims of PPI across the UK can be summarised in the following way:

- Provide patients, carers and the public with opportunities to influence service delivery.
- Create cultures where health professionals actively listen and respond to the views of patients.
- Improve patients' experiences of healthcare and their relationships with clinical professionals.
- Core principles are shared across England, Wales, Scotland and Northern Ireland.
- Provide a statutory duty to consult enshrined in legislation. (British Association of Dermatologists, 2015)

As you can probably see, this is a complex area which requires strong leadership and commitment to the ideals. As a student nurse, it is likely that you will have come across examples of practice where you can clearly see that PPI has had a positive impact on the way in which a service is set up and delivered. Equally, you may have come across situations where this does not seem to be the case. The next section considers how the organisation and culture of clinical practice can impact on the success, or otherwise, of PPI initiatives.

MAKING PPI HAPPEN: THE NEED FOR A NEW STYLE OF LEADERSHIP

A key investigation into NHS leadership and management was undertaken by the King's Fund in 2011. The published report, subtitled *No More Heroes*, argued the case for excellence in leadership and its critical impact on improving patient care. Its main conclusion was that a new style of shared and distributed leadership was needed, not one focused on single heroic individuals, hence the subtitle of the report.

The authors assert that modern leaders are required to work 'through' others and key to their success is the ability to motivate, enthuse and engage 'followers'. Crucially this requires individual leaders to be able to work across different organisations, engaging stakeholders, such as patients and the public, in order to bring about the systemic and transformational change that future successful health systems will require. Following *No More Heroes*, the King's Fund (2012) published a further report about leadership for engagement and improvement in the NHS. It was clear from this critique that engagement matters for both patients and staff because it is seen to transform the experience within the NHS. People who are meaningfully engaged feel respected, listened to and empowered, and are therefore able to influence decisions and consequently improve care.

CULTURE AND POWER

The concepts of culture and power have been discussed in other chapters. You need to consider these concepts and how they promote or inhibit PPI. Failure to do so will arguably leave PPI as a fringe activity.

Culture is a powerful influence on organisations and teams and often manifests in the actions and behaviours of those working within that organisation (Mullins, 2005). Some cultures can be so strong that anyone who does not conform to expected codes of behaviour may be considered an 'outsider' or 'abnormal' and therefore excluded. This is fine when the culture is considered to be positive, as it will encourage a positive behaviour change, but not so good when the prevailing culture is negative or resistant to change. Some 'barometers' that indicate whether a culture is positive include the approach to learning (the learning environment), the way in which staff interact with colleagues, patients and others, and the intangible 'feel' of a clinical area. All of these are important for PPI – it is likely that clinical areas that engage in positive practices in these areas are more likely to take PPI into their practice in meaningful ways.

Activity 5.2

Whilst on clinical placement you may have noticed the prevailing culture, possibly without realising it. You will have observed how clinicians behave, how they talk to each other, how they engage with patients, and the visibility of the leader.

- Is the unit positive about your learning?
- Does the environment feel caring and compassionate?
- Do people make time for you?
- Are people respectful to each other?
- Is there clear leadership?

Take a moment to think through your answers to these questions. The conclusions that you come to will give you an indication of the culture of that particular environment.

Whenever anyone works within a team they will contribute to the culture. It is affected by a whole range of factors, including the values communicated by staff and the attitudes, beliefs and sentiments on display. This is why leadership is important because good leadership sets expectations, models behaviour and promotes a 'desired' culture. Many management theorists have written about culture, perhaps the most famous of whom is Peter Drucker (1999) who talked of culture being critical for success. Drucker argued that a leader can have lots of plans and targets for the team but unless they simultaneously manage and promote the desired culture those plans may take longer to achieve or at worst will fail. Obviously a leader cannot do it alone but must work with teams to shape culture as discussed in *No More Heroes*.

Linked to the concept of culture is the issue of power. Power in the context of nursing and leadership is the capacity to direct or influence the behaviour of others or to influence the course of events. You, as a student nurse, just through your position as a knowledgeable healthcare professional, have power over patients, whether you like that idea or not. Such 'power' can be used as a tool for good – to guide, support and inform – or can be misused – to dominate, undermine or infantilise. Even the use of language such as the term 'my patient' can imply control. Unfortunately, medical terminology is dogged by paternalism that can disempower people and create dependency.

Activity 5.3

In your most recent clinical placement, what language was typically used by the team to refer to patients, their families and team colleagues? Was the language professional and respectful or did it feel uncomfortable? If so, in what way?

The behaviour you display and the language you choose to use to engage in PPI are pivotal because they communicate your values and expectations. You need to consider whether you see the people you engage with as 'equal partners' or 'subservient' in that engagement. If the former, then your efforts to engage will be seen as authentic and valued. If the latter, PPI will be seen as inauthentic and attract accusations of 'tokenism', because whilst you might appear to be seeking shared decision-making, the control and power to decide will remain with you, the professional.

The fundamental principle here for any nurse leader is that if PPI is to be effective health professionals have to firstly address their own attitudes to PPI, and secondly to explore how meaningful patient and public engagement can be exercised to positively influence service provision. If such ideas are applied to nursing leadership in a clinical setting there should, wherever it is possible and safe to do so, be a move away from paternalism (where the health professional takes over) towards joint decision-making: in other words, the aim is to share power. Nurse leaders (and you as a student nurse are already a leader in your own right) are in an ideal position to model good practice and set expectations, to influence the desired culture towards effective PPI, and to impact on shared decision-making.

PPI is certainly the vehicle for ensuring that patients and the public are central to an organisation's mission and purpose. Organisations and individuals within those organisations need to focus on the patient experience and create cultures that provide structures, processes and interactions at all levels that involve patients and the public to achieve greater transparency and address the crisis in public confidence arising from events such as those described in the Francis Report (2013) (Tee, 2012). A useful framework with which to explore these issues is an adaptation of the Manchester Patient Safety Framework (2006) (see Figure 5.1). This can be used to enable health professionals to critically review the cultures of clinical environments in order to move from those that might be considered damaged (pathological), in which patients are largely ignored or seen as an inconvenience, toward cultures where patients and the public are seen as important contributors to the leadership team (generative). By way of illustration in the model in Figure 5.1, organisational cultures can move along a continuum towards increasing maturity from pathological to generative, through three additional developmental phases of 'reactive', 'bureaucratic' and 'proactive'. Although originally developed with a patient safety focus, similar principles apply to developing a PPI culture.

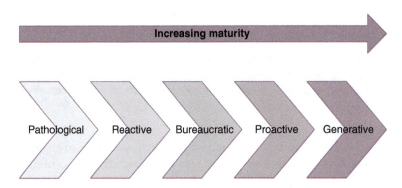

Figure 5.1   A developmental continuum of organisational maturity. (Adapted from the Manchester Patient Safety Framework, 2006)

- Pathological – Why do we need to waste our time on PPI?
- Reactive – We take PPI and do something when we need to.
- Bureaucratic – We have systems in place for PPI.
- Proactive – We are always on the alert/thinking about how PPI can be improved.
- Generative – PPI is an integral part of everything we do.

Movement along this continuum requires leaders to work with their teams and help shape the culture. It's about setting shared values and expectations that patient experience is important and addressing problematic attitudes and assumptions of those in the team. As clinical environments mature and the organisation learns through trying out new approaches to PPI, it will move along the scale toward increasing maturity.

LEADING A MATURE AND GENERATIVE CULTURE OF PPI

To help nurse leaders begin to address cultural issues, a useful study by Luxford and colleagues in 2011 used a number of case studies and data collected from interviews with hospital staff, and patients in hospitals, primary care settings and community-based organisations, to identify factors that were felt to be essential to delivering a high quality patient-oriented service.

The factors they identified were as follows:

1. **Strong and committed senior leadership** to the principles of PPI and patient-centred care – without this it is left to a few champions.
2. **Clear and coherent communication of a strategic vision** that demonstrates commitment to PPI and person-centredness.
3. **Real and authentic engagement** of patients, their families and the wider public in decision-making processes.
4. **A focus on employee satisfaction** – this is important because unhappy and disgruntled staff are less likely to feel inclined to engage. If their own needs go unmet they are less likely to meet others' needs.
5. **A strong emphasis on measurement and feedback** that is reported and acted upon – this ensures the leader is fully aware of what's happening in their clinical environment.
6. **Resourcing for care delivery** – this is where the leader prioritises the necessary resources to deliver patient-centred care.
7. **Building staff capacity to support patient-centred care** – staff need the opportunity to develop and understand PPI. Ongoing CPD (Continuing Professional Development) and staff training is an essential component.
8. **Accountability and incentives** – staff are accountable for their decisions but should also be rewarded for innovation and high quality practice.
9. **Culture supportive of change and learning** – this links to the idea of a 'just' culture, in that opportunities are taken to learn from experience.

Activity 5.4

The list above may appear challenging, and may not seem relevant to you as a student nurse. However, in order to appreciate its relevance to your practice as a student nurse try to:

- Identify one or more of the factors and write down when you have seen such an approach taking place in practice. What was its impact?
- Now consider one of the factors and say how you have (or how you would) take this forward in practice.

'TIME FOR CHANGE'

To further illustrate and enlarge on these issues, work derived from a co-operative inquiry (Tee et al., 2007) involving health service users and staff identified the positive characteristics of a patient and public oriented service. Captured in the 'Time for Change' model, it details 12 essential aspects a leader should address in order to bring about the desired culture.

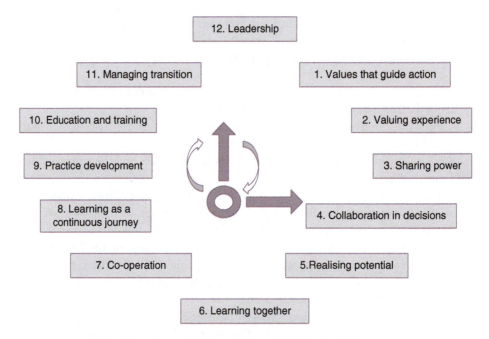

Figure 5.2   'Time for Change' - a model of participation (Tee et al., 2007)

Figure 5.2 illustrates the twelve key elements of the 'Time for Change' model, each of which is described in more detail below.

1. **Values that guide action** – the principles or standards of behaviour that underpin participation in decision-making.
2. **Valuing experience** – the value and recognition of service users' expertise in their own health, and the incorporation of knowledge derived from user-led research into the nurse's decision-making.
3. **Sharing power** – the way in which nurses and other healthcare professionals are vigilant about aspects of their practice which disempower patients either through the use of jargon, or institutional processes which exclude or prevent participation.
4. **Collaboration** – emphasises the humanistic attributes of people working together throughout the care pathway. It seeks to promote greater choice within a client-led framework of care.

5. **Realising potential** – identifies the need to project hope and positive risk-taking that enables the development of confidence and personal responsibility in the support of people's decision-making.

6. **Learning together** – involves service users at the initial planning phases of any aspect of practice, service delivery or evaluation.

7. **Co-operation** – reflects specifically on participants' experience of the process as active agents of change which involves research 'with', rather than 'on', patients/service users.

8. **Learning as a continuous journey** – with opportunities to reflect on practice in order to explore attitudes, values and behaviours; the sharing of experience with patients as a two-way process.

9. **Practice development** – is about facilitating a process of change which leads to cultural transformation. By adopting practice development approaches which embrace a patient-/user-led model, opportunities are created for discussion that challenges practice and promotes understanding.

10. **Education and training** – should employ PPI in the design of courses to promote insights into the lives of service users and themselves as professional carers. The involvement of patients and the public has the potential to reduce the reality gap between theory and practice.

11. **Transition** – is the recognition that services are provided within an environment of constant flux with a need to have systems that maintain an emphasis on the values and philosophy of participation. It is also acknowledged that there will always be people, working within a service, who do not sign up to these values but that their influence should be minimised to ensure continuing and active engagement with the issues.

12. **Leadership** – effective participation is dependent on leadership and management of the clinical environment. This does not mean restrictive bureaucratic procedures, but behaviours which aim to promote a culture of involvement, model participation and recognise difference and individuality.

Activity 5.5

Imagine that you are a member of a team of nurses and that one of your responsibilities is to champion patient and public involvement. Look at the list of activities in the 'Time for Change' model and decide which ones you would implement first. What are the reasons behind your choice? How would you know if you had been successful?

MAKING PPI A REALITY

The King's Fund (2013), in their excellent report on patient leadership, highlight that the most important element in leading PPI is at the level of personal engagement.

This is the most effective way for nurse leaders and managers to see the experience of services through the eyes of the patient. In doing so the nurse leader helps shape both the culture and expectations of practice through appropriate role modelling.

The nurse leader's personal engagement with PPI enables the sharing of power over clinical decisions (Tee et al., 2007) and facilitates a shared dialogue through which the patient can exercise choices and become aware of the benefits, risks and outcomes of potential options. It is evident from studies such as that of Volandes et al. (2011) that, irrespective of background or level of education, the majority of people want to be involved in decisions and clinicians need to find ways of making this happen.

Many of the reported outcomes in recent reports from the Health Ombudsman (2015) in response to patient and public complaints suggest a frequent failure of communication with patients and families. What this suggests is that PPI strategies could enhance practice and avoid such incidents in the future.

Activity 5.6

Now that you have reviewed some of the supporting theories of PPI, make a list of the activities or initiatives that you think could bring about change and enable PPI to be embedded in practice. Once you have done that, decide on *one* thing that you can do in your next clinical placement that relates to one or more of the activities that you have identified (or choose one of the areas identified in Figure 5.3).

You may have thought of some, or all, of the initiatives which are identified in Figure 5.3, which offers some practical examples of methods that have a proven track record of bringing about cultural change.

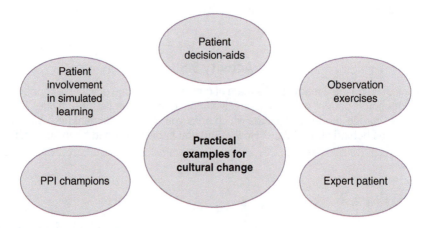

Figure 5.3   Practical examples for cultural change (Tee, 2012)

Working in partnership - Patient Decision Aids (PDAs)

Shared decision-making means 'no decision about me without me'. Typically, patients will come to a decision crossroads where they are faced with a range of alternatives – options to consider. They will often need help to explore these options. One way of doing this is through Patient Decision Aids (PDAs). An organisation called Total Health was engaged by the Rightcare (2012) shared decision-making programme to develop PDAs, published by the BMJ Group. Based on NICE clinical guidelines and clinical quality standards there are over 40 examples.

This PDA gives various options and takes the patient and their family through what the condition is about, the treatment risks, time in hospital, effect on risk, effect on length of life, effect on quality of life, effect of treatment on life and the effect on what you can do. Research has found this to be an extremely valuable process for those facing decision crossroads. It is both patient-led and empowering and when enacted across a service will greatly increase person-centred care.

Expert Patient Initiative

With ever-greater numbers of people coping with a long-term condition, we need to find ways of promoting self-management. The Expert Patient Initiative (NHS Choices, 2014c) derives from the perspective that patients often know their condition better than professionals. However, it is not just about giving patients education, it is also about helping them to develop problem-solving skills and self-efficacy, and facilitating them to apply new knowledge to situations that they may encounter in real-life situations.

We know from research that this initiative improves outcomes and reduces costs. Studies also show that people become more confident, have fewer visits to their doctor, communicate better with professionals, take less time off work and are less likely to require hospital admission (Corrie and Finch, 2015).

Conduct patient leadership walkrounds

Nurse leaders wishing to demonstrate their commitment to PPI and understand the patient experience in their own organisation can do so by making regular leadership rounds with the aim of hearing about the patient experience from patients and staff.

Based on the safety walkrounds work by the Institute for Healthcare Improvement (2000), which specifically focuses on safety, the purpose is to achieve an active two-way dialogue with open and honest sharing and learning. This not only models good practice that communicates to everyone that the 'evidence' from experience is a valid form of feedback, it also influences the culture toward greater openness and transparency, in which everyone feels comfortable sharing examples of good practice and areas of concern.

PPI in simulated learning

A team at Imperial College London led by Professor Roger Kneebone has developed a programme they call 'Reciprocal Illumination', which involves those with expertise through experience (patients and the public) being brought together with people with expertise through professional practice (clinicians) and engaging through simulation activity (Imperial College Centre for Engagement and Simulation Science, 2015).

Patients and staff members re-enact live, or on video, a clinical event which can raise awareness and teach both staff and management valuable lessons. You can tell one true story or patch together real or plausible events to create a fictional composite. A commentary from a senior nurse leader, or the people involved in the real event, can be a powerful ending that reinforces the culture of mutual learning. The most successful are those where everyone involved in an event – including medical staff – contributes to telling the story. You may have experienced such learning in your own university.

Involve patients and the public in new care initiatives

Patients, their families and the wider public are often the best sources of information. Not only do patients and families feel valued when they are involved in new initiatives, but their questions and comments also often indicate where improvements can be made. It is important when conducting such events that the views of patients and their families are taken seriously.

Appoint a PPI champion

Communicating information about patient and public involvement is an important responsibility that should not always fall to managers alone. It is often better to have a staff member in this role. Having a designated PPI champion in every department and patient care unit demonstrates the organisation's commitment to safety and may make other staff members feel more comfortable about sharing information and asking questions. Champions must have proper training, resources and authority.

Conduct observation of patient care experiences

This is purely an exercise in staff setting aside some time to observe the patient's and family's journey through the department. It could not only form a good activity for inducting a new member of staff, it could also be a mechanism for all staff to learn from the patient experience through observation. This learning can then form the basis of an improvement exercise involving the wider team. An example of a helpful observation exercise tool can be found at the Institute for Healthcare Improvement (2014).

Patients as partners in co-design: A service improvement programme

Patients as partners in co-design is an initiative from The Point of Care Foundation (2015) that enables organisations to improve services by working in partnership with patients. They provide several programmes, involving training and coaching by experienced practitioners, using techniques to enable staff to work collaboratively with patients and carers.

As indicated, PPI does not just happen by chance but needs to be championed, supported and nurtured by leaders and managers of healthcare.

For the leader it's as much about the culture and expectations as it is about the systems and processes that let patients have a say. It's also about how leaders grow their teams and encourage patient-centred care and a climate that puts patients at the centre of decision-making. To summarise what needs to be done you can look at the King's Fund (2013) publication (*Patient-Centred Leadership – Rediscovering Our Purpose*) that suggests leaders in healthcare need to routinely act on patient feedback and hear patient stories, involve patients in developing a culture in which their needs come first, facilitate openness and honesty amongst their teams and ensure patient-centred care is understood at all levels of the organisation. Only when we see this level of commitment will PPI become central to health service delivery rather than a fringe activity.

SUMMARY

This chapter has sought to highlight the importance of the student nurse understanding, engaging and moving forward with the PPI agenda.

Some key points include:

- Patient and public involvement is an important component of effective healthcare leadership.
- Effective patient and public involvement is dependent on creating a culture that recognises its value.
- The degree of patient and public involvement can be an important indicator of patient-centred care.

FURTHER RESOURCES

The 'Patients' Voices' website aims to put patients' experiences at the centre of healthcare. The website provides access to numerous learning resources including videos of patients talking about their experiences: www.patientvoices.org.uk

The British Association of Dermatologists website is an excellent professional site offering access to a whole range of resources to support PPI: www.bad.org.uk/healthcare-professionals/clinical-services/patient-and-public-involvement

Watch Brian and Ruth's interviews on the companion website at https://study.sagepub.com/taylor to find out more about their experiences of being nurse leaders.

REFERENCES

British Association of Dermatologists (2015) *Public and Patient Information*. [Online] Available at: www.bad.org.uk/healthcare-professionals/clinical-services/patient-and-public-involvement. Accessed 31/08/15.

Corrier, C. and Finch, A. (2015) *Expert Patients*. London: Reform Research Trust.

Department of Health (2000) *The NHS Plan: A Plan for Investment, a Plan for Reform*. [Online] Available at http://webarchive.nationalarchives.gov.uk/+/www.dh.gov.uk/en/publicationsandstatistics/publications/publicationspolicyandguidance/dh_4002960. Accessed 31/08/15.

Department of Health (2008) *The Next Stage Review*. London: Office of Public Sector Information.

Department of Health (2009) *The NHS Constitution for England*. London: DH. [Online] Available at https://www.gov.uk/government/publications/the-nhs-constitution-for-england. Accessed 27/05/16.

Department of Health (2010) *Equity and Excellence: Liberating the NHS*. London: Office of Public Sector Information.

Drucker, P. (1999) *Management Challenges for the 21st Century*. London: Elsevier.

Edwards, A.G.K., Naik, G., Ahmed, H., Elwyn, G.J., Pickles, T., Hood, K. and Playle, R. (2013) *Personalised Risk Communication for Informed Decision Making about Taking Screening Tests*. Cochrane Review.

Francis, R. (2013) *The Mid Staffordshire Public Inquiry*. [Online] Available at www.midstaffspublicinquiry.com. Accessed 31/08/15.

Health Ombudsman (2015) Health Reports 2014/15. [Online] Available at www.ombudsman.org.uk/reports-and-consultations/reports/health. Accessed 19/02/2016.

Imperial College Centre for Engagement and Simulation Science (2015) *Reciprocal Illumination*. [Online] Available at http://www3.imperial.ac.uk/newsandeventspggrp/imperialcollege/medicine/newssummary/news_20-2-2013-15-52-50. Accessed 31/08/15.

Institute for Healthcare Improvement (2000) *Patient Safety Leadership WalkRounds*. Cambridge: MA: Institute for Healthcare Improvement Idealized Design Group and Allan Frankel, MD.

Institute for Healthcare Improvement (2014) *Patient Care Experience Observation Exercise*. [Online] Available at www.ihi.org/resources/Pages/Tools/PatientCareExperienceObservationExercise.aspx. Accessed 31/08/15.

King's Fund (2011) *The Future of leadership and Management in the NHS: No More Heroes*. Report from The King's Fund Commission on Leadership and Management in the NHS. London: Kings Fund.

King's Fund (2012) *Leadership and Engagement for Improvement in the NHS: Together We Can*. Report from The King's Fund Leadership Review. London: King's Fund.

King's Fund (2013) *Patient Centred Leadership:Rediscovering our purpose*. London: King's Fund. Available at www.kingsfund.org.uk/sites/files/kf/field/field_publication_file/patient-centred-leadership-rediscovering-our-purpose-may13.pdf. Accessed 31/08/15.

Lloyd, M. (2010) 'Participation in practice: a review of service user involvement in mental health nursing'. *Mental Health and Learning Disability Research and Practice*, 7: 195–207.

Luxford, K., Gelb Safran, D., Delbanco, T. (2011) 'Promoting patient-centered care: a qualitative study of facilitators and barriers in healthcare organizations with a reputation for improving the patient experience'. *International Journal for Quality in Health Care*. [Online] Available at http://intqhc.oxfordjournals.org/content/23/5/510. Accessed 31/08/15.

Manchester Patient Safety Framework (MaPSaF) (2006) [Online] Available at www.nrls.npsa.nhs.uk/resources. Accessed 31/08/15.

Mullins, L.J. (2005) *Management and Organisational Behaviour*, 7th edition. London: Prentice Hall.

NHS Choices (2014a) *NHS Constitution*. [Online] Available at www.nhs.uk/choiceintheNHS/Rightsandpledges/NHSConstitution/Pages/Overview.aspx. Accessed 31/08/15.

NHS Choices (2014b) *NHS Choices Framework* [Online] Available at www.nhs.uk/Pages/HomePage.aspx. Accessed 31/08/15.

NHS Choices (2014c) *Expert Patient Programme*. [Online] Available at www.nhs.uk/NHSEngland/AboutNHSservices/doctors/Pages/expert-patients-programme.aspx. Accessed 31/08/15.

NHS Northern Ireland (2011) *Personal and Public Involvement (PPI) Public Health Agency*. [Online] Available at: http://www.publichealth.hscni.net/directorate-nursing-and-allied-health-professions/allied-health-professions-and-personal-and-publi-5. Accessed 07/06/16.

NHS Wales (2015) *Patient Experience*. [Online] Available at www.wales.nhs.uk/sites3/home.cfm?orgid=420. Accessed 31/08/15.

Patient and Public Involvement Solutions (2012) *Putting People at the Heart of Public Services*. [Online] Available at www.patientpublicinvolvement.com. Accessed 31/08/15.

Point of Care Foundation (2015) *Patients as Partners in Co-design*. [Online] Available at www.pointofcarefoundation.org.uk/What-We-Do. Accessed 31/08/15.

Rightcare (2012) *Patient Decision Aids – NHS Shared Decision Making*. [Online] Available at http://sdm.rightcare.nhs.uk. Accessed 31/08/15.

Scottish Government (2011) Patient Rights (Scotland) Act 2011. The Scottish Government. Available at www.gov.scot/Home#slide/1 . Accessed 07/06/16.

Stringer, B., Van Meijel, B., De Vree, W. and Van Der Bijl, J. (2008) 'User involvement in mental health care: the role of nurses: a literature review'. *Journal of Psychiatric and Mental Health Nursing*, 15: 678–83.

Tadd, W., Hillman, A., Calnan, S., Calnan, M., Bayer, T. and Read, S. (2011) 'Dignity in practice: an exploration of the care of older adults in acute NHS trusts'. NIHR Service Delivery and Organisation Programme. Project 08/1819/218. Southampton: NETSCC – SDO.

Tee S.R. (2012) 'Service user involvement – addressing the crisis in confidence in healthcare'. Editorial. *Nurse Education Today*. DOI: 10.1016/j.nedt.2011.12.002. [Online] Available at http://dx.doi.org/10.1016/j.nedt.2011.12.002. Accessed 31/08/15.

Tee, S., Lathlean, J., Herbert, L., Coldham, T., East, B. and Johnson, T-J. (2007) 'User participation in mental health nurse decision-making: a co-operative enquiry'. *Journal of Advanced Nursing*, 60(2): 135–45.

Volandes, A.E., Ferguson, L.A., Davis, A.D., Hull, N.C., Green, M.J., Chang, Y., Deep, K. and Paasche-Orlow, M.K. (2011) 'Assessing end-of-life preferences for advanced dementia in rural patients using an educational video: a randomized controlled trial'. *Journal of Palliative Medicine*, 14: 169–77.

Wetzels, R., Harmsen, M., Van Weel, C., Grol, R. and Wensing, M. (2007) 'Interventions for improving older patients' involvement in primary care episodes', *Cochrane Database Syst Rev*. 2007;(1):CD004273 [PubMed].

6 GLOBAL ISSUES FOR NURSING LEADERSHIP

Mary Gobbi

Chapter learning outcomes

On completion of this chapter you will be able to:

- Explain how globalisation and migration issues impact upon patients, staff, healthcare needs and health services.
- Identify how changing patterns of disease can have a global impact on the role of nurse leaders.
- Describe how different modes of healthcare, healthcare regulation and healthcare education affect the mobility of nurses.
- Identify issues that clinical and executive leaders need to consider when operating in a global context.

Key concepts

Globalisation, cultural competence, migration, regulation, international health

---

INTRODUCTION

In this chapter, I hope to inspire you with some of the challenges, intrigues and joys of leading and working within, and across, different countries and cultures. Many of you are already working with care assistants, registered nurses and other healthcare professionals who have lived, and in some cases qualified, in other countries. Similarly, I expect that you have encountered patients, families and carers who have also spent all, or part, of their lives, in another country. Some of you may be making plans to have a student experience aboard, or to work abroad following registration. Perhaps you have come to the UK to gain your qualifications here. This chapter will help you to understand why people move, what health challenges emerge, and what skills and competences executive nurse leaders need so that they can plan their services to cater for new migrations of patients and staff.

As I write this chapter, the news is full of examples of the mass movement of people seeking better places to live and work, whether it be from Africa and the Middle East to Europe, Mexico to the United States of America, or South East Asia to Australia (BBC News Channel, nd). As people move, they carry their existing health challenges from their country of origin (COA), and then encounter those of their new country – the host/ destination country. In 2014 the world faced the Ebola crisis and some nurses went to work in Central Africa to offer their expertise. Regretfully, some came back with Ebola. Scottish nurse Pauline Cafferkey was one of those people and she was much in the news at the time (for example: www.scotsman.com/news/scots-ebola-nurse-pauline-cafferkey-is-improving-1–3658456). This movement of people, whether as recipients of healthcare and/or providers of healthcare, is a direct consequence of the process of globalisation.

The chapter starts by reviewing the term 'globalisation' and what factors encourage or deter people from moving countries. The second part of the chapter considers what it means to be a registered nurse and leader in a multicultural society. You therefore need to understand how culture, demography and public health trends influence service provision, beliefs about health and care and the role of the nurse leader. I refer to you as a student nurse leader in this chapter – remember that a key thread across this book is the student nurse as leader. It doesn't mean that you will necessarily be responsible for all the areas that I discuss in this chapter. But you do need to have knowledge of the issues and will soon be taking responsibility for these areas as a qualified nurse.

The chapter then reflects on the issues that arise when staff are mobile and immigrate or emigrate. This relates to the ways in which regulations and the nursing scope of practice differ from country to country. Throughout the chapter the implications of these factors for nurse leaders today and tomorrow are analysed. Let's start with the concept of globalisation.

GLOBALISATION

Globalisation is a process that describes the way in which people and countries are increasingly connected and interdependent. Globalisation occurs when barriers to movement are reduced and people, goods, money, services and ideas move from one part of the world to another and cross national boundaries. Technology can enhance globalisation through swift and 'real time' communications that enable quick dissemination of information and the rapid spread of news, ideas and data. Therefore, globalisation causes changes in economic activity, politics, social and cultural development, and technology (adapted from the World Health Organization (WHO), 2015).

Any definition of globalisation refers to the movement of people and 'things' between countries. Figure 6.1 summarises some of the factors that influence healthcare and nursing in a globalised world.

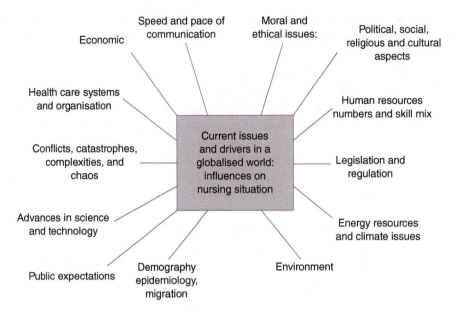

Figure 6.1   Global factors that influence health care and nursing

Many of the factors identified within Figure 6.1 interact with one another to generate what are called 'push and pull' factors in the movement of people from one country to another (Kline, 2003). Typical 'push' factors are those associated with poverty, natural disasters like droughts or floods, war, conflict, persecution and government strategies to encourage their population to move. 'Pull' factors are things like open borders, the ability to physically move, economic or lifestyle rewards, and job vacancies. Specifically within the context of health services, people may move temporarily (health tourism) or permanently to ensure that their health is improved, treated or maintained when the services in the host country are more accessible and/or of higher quality than in their home country. Further information on how the movement of patients across borders presents public health challenges can be found in Helbe (2010) on the WHO website if you are interested in exploring this issue further.

Activity 6.1

Have you encountered any instances of health tourism? How did it make you feel? Does it matter if health tourism is undertaken privately (the person pays for it) or covertly (the person comes to the country intentionally to avoid paying and does not declare this)?

Sometimes staff report that it seems unfair that someone has, apparently, deliberately come to the UK, presented as an 'emergency in the NHS' and then received treatment, while a local person may have apparently had to 'wait' their turn. As a student nurse, it is certainly your responsibility to understand the entitlements to 'free access', so that you can notify the relevant administration staff should payment be appropriate. Whatever the 'rights and wrongs' of a situation, if someone requires treatment, they should be treated impartially as outlined in the Nursing and Midwifery Council Code (NMC, 2015).

Nurse leaders also need to be aware of wider political initiatives that can potentially influence nurses, nursing and patient care. Health provision and services also feature as part of national and international trade agreements. One example of this is the Transatlantic Trade and Investment Partnership (TTIP) – which you may have read about in the news. At the time of writing, the European Union (EU) and the United States of America (US) are negotiating a new trade agreement that is designed to create a more flexible market between the EU and the US. It is unclear how the 2016 EU Referendum outcome will impact on TTIP. Historically, the National Health Service (NHS) has been excluded from such agreements. There is concern that the negotiations, which are largely held in secret, will no longer exempt health services from the agreement, meaning that the NHS may be opened up to American private business. For further information you can look at the Royal College of Nursing international work web page: www.rcn.org.uk/international.

It is important that you are aware of the global issues affecting healthcare, and the impact that possible changes such as the one described here may have on your practice.

Activity 6.2

What is your opinion on the potential inclusion of health services within the TTIP? Why? Whatever your view, how could you make your voice heard?

Modern communications have a globalising effect. For example, with telemedicine the client and/or their data can be accessed and their medical data analysed from another country. Originally, this would have occurred from an area of high resource/ expertise to one without. To enable such borders to be crossed, infrastructures need to be in place and the technology must be useable and of low cost for the developing area. Appropriate regulations and legal frameworks also need to be in place. Patient confidentiality and the security of data are typical challenges. For transnational partnership to work, Saliba et al.'s (2012) study found that strong leadership was crucial. This sharing of resources to cut costs within and between countries was not only predicted (Robinson et al., 2003), but has also now occurred (for example with the transfer of radiological images and web-based cameras used by the military in conflict zones).

Another area where web-based communications have increasing importance is in the management of disasters. For example, you could use 'crowdsourcing' to find ways to deliver supplies. Crowdsourcing is a technique where internet-based communications are used to access the talent and resources of large numbers of people to achieve a set, often time-limited, goal. One example of where 'big data' and crowdsourcing were used in a disaster situation is provided in case study 6.1.

Case study 6.1: Big data – Nepal earthquake

Researchers from the Universities of Southampton, Oxford and Nottingham collaborated with rescue agencies to provide 'real time' information at the time of the Nepal earthquake in 2015. Using sophisticated mapping techniques they identified priority areas for water filters. Crowdsourcing techniques enabled them to plot the movement of peoples and where they settled so that resources could be targeted specifically by the local and international aid agencies. (See: www.orchid.ac.uk/presses/orchid-researchers-provide-nepal-earthquake-response.)

Huynen et al. (2005) provide an example of how globalisation has health impacts. The researchers identified the main determinants or features of population health and globalisation and then constructed a model. They concluded that population health was influenced at many levels by various interacting factors including, at a general level, the institutional frameworks and the economic, social–cultural and environmental (eco-logical) determinants of public health. Specifically, while globalisation mainly works at the infrastructural or contextual level, its impact on health is associated with more practical issues related to the basic environment, social and knowledge lifestyles, trade mechanisms, policies and services. This means that nursing assessments need to address these practical factors when patients and staff move from one country to another. As a student nurse with a growing knowledge-base, you should ensure that you use this knowledge appropriately *now* and not wait until you are qualified if there are times when you can influence care positively.

INTERNATIONAL HEALTH ISSUES

There are various sources of data to help us understand global health challenges. The annual WHO Report points out general trends. The most recent report gives data from 2014 (WHO, 2014) revealing that across the world, deaths from measles have been cut by nearly 80% since 2000, that nearly 800 women die every day due to preg-nancy and childbirth, and that a child born in Africa is eight times more likely to die before their fifth birthday than a child born in the EU. This same report noted that the three top causes of premature death are ischaemic heart disease, lower respiratory tract infections and stroke. However, there are variations according to the countries under analysis. So, for Organisation for Economic Co-Operation and Development countries (OECD, 2013) (see information box 6.1 for an overview of the OECD), two of the top causes of disease are the same as those in the WHO (2014) report (ischae-mic heart disease and stroke), but the third is cancer, with suicide being a significant cause of death. The mortality rate for some diseases (e.g. stroke) is reducing in OECD countries with higher survival rates for other diseases (e.g. cancer). It is also important to recognise that some countries have cultural practices that give rise to specific health risks and problems, for example female genital mutilation (FGM) and beliefs about mental health illness.

Your awareness of the particular health risks associated with a person's country of origin means that you can ensure that nursing assessments sensitively include reference to these risks. In some cases, you may find that staff (or you) require specific education and training, perhaps in culturally sensitive communication (in the case of FGM or suspected mental illness) or a particular nursing technique (urinary catheterisation). However, strategically you need to consider the probability of meeting individuals with these health challenges through your awareness of local population statistics and demography.

Information box 6.1: The Organisation for Economic Co-operation and Development

The Organisation for Economic Co-Operation and Development (OECD) comprises 34 subscribing countries. It was established after World War Two to promote peace through reconstruction and co-operation between countries. Its goal is to build a stronger, fairer world. The OECD monitors developments and activities within its members, compares and contrasts their data and makes recommendations to improve the economic performance of both the member countries and the world economy. The member countries are largely developed countries, but emerging (India and Brazil) and developing countries in Africa and Asia can become members.

It is important to identify whether people from different cultures, ethnicities and countries hold similar beliefs about the cause and treatment of their illness. I have been associated with a stream of research investigating the extent to which Cognitive Behavioural Therapy (CBT) needs adaptation according to the ethnicity, culture and location of the client. For example when working with colleagues (Naeem et al., 2014) we found that CBT not only needed cultural adaptation, but that patients and their carers in Pakistan also sought help from a variety of sources. They used a bio-psycho-spiritual-social model of illness. To illustrate this, a client might attribute the cause of their psychosis to 'something in the air', 'chemicals in my brain' or magic. You can probably see from this one example that it is essential you understand the needs of different communities and the impact these differences have on your leadership of clinical practice. To take this discussion one step further, and to provide you with some further materials to fuel your thinking about health issues in a global context, information box 6.2 provides some facts and figures about the topic.

Information box 6.2: Global facts and figures

- The countries with the lowest life expectancy (which means the years someone can expect to live from the moment they are born) are Chad, Central African Republic and Angola (WHO, 2014).
- There is a rising epidemic of childhood obesity, including in Africa (WHO, 2014).
- Nearly one in two adult men consume tobacco in the WHO Western Pacific region (WHO, 2014).
- There are concerns over the inadequate number of doctors qualified to work in primary care (OECD, 2013).
- There are concerns in many countries about a shortage of nurses and an aging nursing workforce. High-income countries have on average more nurses and midwives per 10,000 people than low-income countries – an average ratio of 90:2 (OECD, 2013).
- More than 15% of people (mainly women) aged 50 and older provide care for a dependent relative or friend (OECD, 2013).
- Due to the economic recession, many countries (e.g. Greece, Iceland) are spending less on health, especially health prevention expenditure (OECD, 2013).

Activity 6.3

Feel free to explore the websites where these facts and figures come from. Data from the WHO are usually at the regional level and can be found at: www.who.int/gho/publications/world_health_statistics/2014/en.

The OECD presents detailed comparisons for member countries: http://stats.oecd.org/index.aspx?DataSetCode=HEALTH_STAT.

Consider what these data might mean for the provision of health services within and between countries. You could also think about how one or more of the issues are affecting your work as a nurse – for example, the rise in mental health problems and the increasing prevalence of obesity.

As I have alluded to, the inevitable outcome of migration is that healthcare providers and professionals need to consider cultural issues in all aspects of their work. Leaders must demonstrate a multicultural and diverse approach, or 'transcultural care' (Northouse, 2010). As I have shown, when people move, they bring with them their existing health challenges, values, beliefs and experiences and then they may acquire and encounter those of the host country. To understand this further, we need to be able to distinguish between the legal status of individuals and their human rights as people deserving dignity and respect.

In 1951, the United Nations High Commissioner for Refugees (UNHCR) produced a Refugee Convention (Article 1 para A1 and A2). This Convention stated clearly that a refugee is someone who:

owing to a well-founded fear of being persecuted for reasons of race, religion, nationality, membership of a particular social group or political opinion, is outside the country of his nationality, and is unable to, or owing to such fear, is unwilling to avail himself of the protection of that country.

These terms are defined in international law.

The terms asylum-seeker and refugee are often confused: an asylum-seeker is someone who says he or she is a refugee, but whose claim has not yet been confirmed. According to the UNHCR website (2015), on average about one million people seek asylum on an individual basis every year. Refugees are people who cross international borders to seek security and sanctuary. They have human and legal rights under international law, including the right not to be returned home while it remains dangerous with potentially deadly consequences. The most vulnerable group are internally displaced people (IDP). They are people who have left their homes within their home country typically due to conflict, violence or persecution. Their legal protection rests with their government, even though the government itself may be the cause of their problems. In contrast, migrants are people who have chosen to move country for other reasons, for example economic benefit, to improve their lives or to live with other family members. Migrants can normally return home safely. This next definition of migration summarises the key issues for healthcare practitioners.

> Migration is a process of moving, either across an international border, or within a state. It is a population movement, encompassing any kind of movement of people, whatever its length, composition and cause. Migration health addresses the state of physical, mental and social wellbeing of migrants and mobile populations. The structural inequalities experienced by many migrants have a significant impact on overall health and wellbeing. Migration health thus goes beyond the traditional management of diseases among mobile populations and is intrinsically linked with the broader social determinants of health and unequal distribution of such determinants. (Davies et al., 2010: 10).

Once again, we see how crucial the nursing assessment is. It must cover the broader social determinants of health through sensitive observation and questioning of the person's lifestyle, beliefs and background.

Activity 6.4

In the context of healthcare, find definitions for the following terms and give a practical example of how the concept is important to your leadership in practice by referring to the NMC Code (2015):

- Multiculturalism.
- Diversity.
- Ethnocentricity.
- Prejudice and stereotyping.

Familiarity with these concepts means that you can take active steps to prevent discrimination and inequalities from arising. For example, prejudice can arise when people make statements about groups of people that are inaccurate, and lead to them being treated with suspicion, fear, or being denied choice in their treatment or management. Services that are designed for one race, culture or ethnicity may not be appropriate for another. It is your responsibility to gather the facts, find out what people really believe, think and desire and then collaboratively help plan the nursing care. Similarly, if you hear evidence of discrimination, ethnocentricity or inequity, then you should take steps to report this and prevent it from escalating further. Do you know who you would report this to in your clinical placements?

While all people, irrespective of status, should be treated with respect and dignity and their human rights upheld, the legal rights of the individual depend upon their status as migrant, refugee, asylum seeker or displaced person. Broadly speaking, refugees and asylum seekers have protection under international law, internally displaced persons are subject to the rules of their home country, while migrants are subject to the laws and policies of their destination country. This is why it is essential to know the legal status of the person. However, you should consider the issues from an ethical perspective: what duties and responsibilities do nurses and healthcare workers have towards the individual person who is unwell or injured?

Activity 6.5

Consider the following scenario, apply the Code of Practice, and discuss what you think the nursing actions should be.

> Scenario – You are working in the emergency department and someone is admitted who claims to be an asylum seeker. Their English language is poor, and the person appears to have an acute, life threatening, abdominal complaint.

Question 1: Are they entitled to prompt treatment for their abdominal complaint? What would your nursing actions be?

Question 2: Would your response be the same if they were: (a) a migrant; (b) an EU citizen; (c) a non-EU holiday maker.

Question 3: With respect to the people listed above what is your duty of care irrespective of the funding issue?

Question 4: Of the people listed in Question 2, are any of them required, in the UK, to pay for their treatment? What factors determine this?

Answers to activity 6.5

- Questions 1 and 2: All these people are entitled to be treated in the same way, in that they have a life threatening condition.

> ○   Actions you take should include: treating the clinical situation as an abdominal emergency with all the associated nursing actions. For the client in the scenario and potentially for the non-EU holiday maker (depending on their English language skills) it is important to arrange an interpreter as soon as possible. Determining capacity for their consent may be problematic if there is a language barrier and the person cannot understand the staff. However, you can liaise with the medical and governance staff of the hospital (and any language competent relatives who have the patient's consent), so that the team can 'act in the best interests' of the client.
>
> • Question 3: Your duty of care is the same to each person, as the NMC Code (2015) outlines, particularly the Prioritising People Section 1 'Treat people as individuals and uphold their dignity' and Section 4 'Acting in the best interests of people at all times'.
> • Question 4: Payment for NHS services received does depend upon the person's circumstances and the criteria may change from time to time. Always check this with your finance department. At the time of writing, the non-EU holiday maker on a visitor visa, should expect to be charged for their NHS treatment, with their holiday insurance usually covering the costs. Migrants may be required to pay an 'immigration healthcare surcharge' as part of their application. They can then use the NHS. If the asylum seeker has been granted refugee status, or made an application for temporary protection, then they can access the NHS in the usual way. Most people who live or work in another European Economic Area country and from Switzerland can get free NHS care if they use their European Health Insurance Card (EHIC). The NHS can then reclaim the costs from the issuing country. There are some exceptions to this rule relating to a person's ability to work and their entitlement to have an EHIC.

It is important to understand what specific public health challenges are encountered by migrants. A review of the situation within the EU is provided by Weekers et al. (2009). In this report they identify that migrants may:

• delay seeking care due to different beliefs about illness;
• have different perceptions about the role of healthcare staff (e.g. midwives and nurses);
• use traditional healers or herbs and then not share this information;
• have health problems that are not typical, not funded or not resourced, in their destination country;
• experience discrimination.

As these examples demonstrate, healthcare professionals may need to rethink the way they organise and deliver care. Weekers et al. (2009) argue for a transformed health workforce with new competencies that have particular relevance for nurse leaders and include training in intercultural competence, an open-mindedness to different models of healthcare, and the ability to learn about the health conditions of migrants, epidemiology and rights to healthcare. As a student nurse and aspiring leader, what this means is that you need to learn how to communicate with, and actively listen, to the needs of clients from different cultures. During your nursing programme you will have had education on diversity and equality, but how does this relate to your clients? Do you know the ethnic, religious and socio-economic and cultural make up of your local population? Are there belief systems with which you are unfamiliar? If this is the case then devise a personal learning plan to familiarise yourself with these populations and their specific needs. Consider how you can demonstrate to clients respect for their values, needs and traditions, while working with them to improve their health and wellbeing and design care plans that are suited to their way of life.

NURSE MIGRATION

Globalisation can lead to movement of the labour force, in this case nurses and other healthcare professionals who respond to the 'push and pull' factors that influence mobility. Nurse migration can be a contentious topic being associated with ethical issues of recruitment (if rich countries recruit from poorer countries and leave the poorer countries without staff); thorny challenges of patient safety (what language and cultural competence is required when in a host country?); and how to manage any potential differences in the standards and scope of practice between home and host country. The key issues for international nurse recruitment are summarised by the Royal College of Nursing (2002), the Department of Health has a UK Code of Practice for International Recruitment (2004) and NHS Scotland produced their Code in 2006. Many other countries draw on the WHO Codes, with the most recent being published in 2010.

When preparing an induction for migrant nurses, you need to consider what might be significant country differences in mechanisms of financing, how the profession is regulated, the roles of professional associations, codes and scope of practice, practice standards, evidence-based practice, professional values, issues of revalidation, and experiences of education and training. The nurse leader has a responsibility to do a training needs analysis with the migrant nurse, taking these factors into account. A learning and development plan can then be implemented and evaluated, sensitive to the talents and skills of the nurse as well any knowledge or skill gaps that need attention.

QUALITIES OF NURSE LEADERS IN A GLOBAL CONTEXT

Kulwicki (2006) argues that it is necessary to have a global perspective to nursing practice, education and research through the development of culturally diverse and responsive models of care. Furthermore, it is becoming increasingly important that nurse leaders engage with the political processes. For example, Gobbi (2014) and De Raeve

(2011) have shown how the political leadership of nurses in Europe has led to changes in the nursing legislation that have improved patient safety (e.g. language testing). Several authors and studies have recommended competences of nurse leaders to enable them to be ready for the emerging world of 2020. One example is the work of the EU/US Atlantis Project in which a three-country study (the US, the UK and Germany) was conducted to identify key benchmarks for global nurse leaders. The key benchmarks were clustered under the following headings:

- Moral and ethical agency.
- (Inter)personal qualities.
- Strategic and systems skills.
- Knowledge management and decision-making skills.
- Patient safety.
- Workforce development.
- Quality improvement.

Further details can be found on the University of Washington, Seattle, website (http://collaborate.uw.edu/tools-and-curricula/global-nursing-leadership-toolkit.html).

Activity 6.6

Take one or more of these headings and using the scope of practice implied within the Code (NMC, 2015), identify an area for your personal development plan as a future leader in a global context. Consider the ways in which you will develop your skills and knowledge in these areas, and make a plan to take forward at least one area for your own personal and professional development. Here are a few examples:

NMC Code reference and issue	Self audit/action plan
Always practise in line with best available evidence (Section 6). Benchmark competence: Patient safety What is the make up of our local population, do I know their needs?	Has there been an audit in my clinical area with respect to meeting the needs of clients from X population? If not, find out whether there is an audit tool available, and/or design one with the community. As a leader, I need to develop an action plan based on the outcomes of the audit.
Recognise and work within the limits of your competence (Section 13). Benchmark statement: Moral and ethical agency. From a leadership perspective, how do I handle difficult conversations with staff who may be showing unconscious prejudice? Do I need some training?	Identify training opportunities through dialogue with the diversity officers. Find out ways to detect signs of unconscious prejudice or bias in your staff.

Nurse leaders are facing many challenges in an often unpredictable world. In contrast, ready access to international communications, debates, data and peoples offers unprecedented opportunities to network, collaborate and learn from others in the global nursing community and with other disciplines. You will read more about this in Chapter 8 (Networking and leadership). I have been privileged to travel extensively and work with colleagues in different countries, whether rich or poor economically. Wherever one works, the patient still faces their health challenges within the context of the culture, country and resources available. Similarly, nursing colleagues operate within their scope of practice, culture, context and resources. What we share is a passion for people that transcends boundaries, yet requires sensitive, morally strong and committed nurse leaders willing to strive for the best for all peoples.

SUMMARY

Some key points from this chapter are:

- Nurse leaders must be sensitive to the changing public health needs of the population, paying attention to new patterns of disease, epidemiology, demography and the movement of peoples.
- Leaders must initiate new models of care, and be prepared to innovate and lead a multicultural workforce serving increasingly diverse populations.
- To be equipped to lead in 2020, in an ever-increasingly technological, web-based, chaotic and conflict-ridden world, leaders need new skills and competences. In particular they need skills in complex transcultural decision-making; handling sensitive political processes; and maintaining sound moral and ethical values when challenged by adverse circumstances, financial constraints, conflicts and threats to patient safety.

FURTHER RESOURCES

The WHO Annual Reports provide data on the global and country-based trends in health, the health workforce, disease patterns and initiatives. See www.who.int/publications/en.

The International Council of Nurses (www.icn.ch) works to improve conditions for both patients and nurses at a global level. Their website contains many interesting policies, procedures and news. In addition, their journal, *International Nursing Review*, has articles from different parts of the world.

Information on female genital mutilation: www.who.int/reproductivehealth/topics/fgm/prevalence/en.

The ICN Burdett Global Nursing Leadership Institute was founded in 2009 to provide leadership education and training for senior and executive nurses. http://leadership.icn.ch/gnli/

The Nuffield Trust talks: a range of topics of interest for leaders www.nuffieldtrust.org.uk/talks/slideshows/rebecca-rosen-trends-and-drivers-change-primary-care.

To access further resources related to this chapter, please visit the companion website at https://study.sagepub.com/taylor

Country databases and information

European Union: www.euro.who.int/en/who-we-are/partners/observatory.

OECD (2015) *Health at a Glance 2015: OECD Indicators*. Paris, PECD Publishing. DOI: http://dx.doi.org/10.1787/health_glance-2015-en

World Bank: http://data.worldbank.org/data-catalog/world-development-indicators.

WHO: www.who.int/gho/publications/world_health_statistics/2014/en.

REFERENCES

BBC News Channel (nd) http://news.bbc.co.uk/1/shared/spl/hi/world/04/migration/html/migration_boom.stm. Accessed 30/11/15.

Davies, A.D., Basten, A. and Frattini, C. (2010) 'Migration: A social determinant of migrants' health'. *Eurohealth*, 16(1): 10–12.

De Raeve, P. (2011) *Nurses' Voice in the EU Policy Process*. Belgium: Kluwer.

Department of Health (2004) *Code of Practice for NHS Employers Involved in the International Recruitment of Healthcare Professionals*. London: DH.

Gobbi, M. (2014) 'Nursing leadership in the European landscape: influence, reality and politics'. *Journal of Nursing Research*, 19(7–8): 636–46. DOI: 10.1177/1744987114557109.

Helbe, M. (2010) 'The movement of patients across borders: challenges and opportunities for public health'. *Bulletin of the World Health Organization*, 89: 68–72. DOI: 10.2471/BLT.10.076612 www.who.int/bulletin/volumes/89/1/10-076612/en. Accessed 12/9/2016.

Huynen, M.M.T.E., Martens, P. and Hilderink, H.B.M. (2005) 'The health impacts of globalisation: a conceptual framework'. *Globalization and Health*, 1:14. DOI: 10.1186/1744-8603-1-14.

Kline, D.S. (2003) 'Push and pull factors in international nurse migration'. *Journal of Nursing Scholarship*, 35: 107–11. DOI: 10.1111/j.1547-5069.2003.00107.

Kulwicki, A. (2006) 'Improving global health care through diversity'. *Journal of Transcultural Nursing*, 17(4): 396–7.

Naeem, F., Habib, N., Gul, M., Khalid, M. et al. (2014) 'A qualitative study to explore patients', carers', and health professionals' views to culturally adapt CBT for psychosis in Pakistan (CBTp)'. *Behavioural and Cognitive Psychotherapy*, 2: 1–13. DOI: http://dx.doi.org/10.1017/S1352465814000332.

NHS Scotland. (2006) *Code of Practice for the International Recruitment of Healthcare Professionals in Scotland*. Edinburgh: Scottish Executive.

Northouse, P.G. (2010) *Leadership: Theory and Practice*, 5th edition. London: Sage.

Nursing and Midwifery Council. (2015) *The Code: Professional Standards of Practice and Behaviour for Nurses and Midwives*. London: NMC.

OECD (2013) *Health at a Glance 2013: OECD Indicators*. Paris: OECD. DOI: http://dx.doi.org/10.1787/health_glance-2013-sum-en

Robinson, D., Savage, G.T. and Campbell, K.S. (2003) 'Organizational learning, diffusion of innovation, and international collaboration'. *Health Care Management Review*, 28(1): 68–72.

Royal College of Nursing (2002) *Internationally Recruited Nurses: Good Practice Guidance for Health Care Employers and RCN Negotiators*. London: RCN.

Saliba, V., Legido-Quigley, H., Hallik, R., Aaviksoo, A., Car, J. and McKee, M. (2012) 'Telemedicine across borders: a systematic review of factors that hinder or support implementation'. *International Journal of Medical Informatics*, 81(12): 793–809. DOI: 10.1016/j.ijmedinf.2012.08.003.

UNHCR (1951) *Convention and Protocol Relating to the Status of Refugees*. Text of the 1951 Convention Relating to the Status of Refugees, Chapter 1, page 14.

UNHCR (2015) [Online] *UNHCR viewpoint: 'refugee' or 'migrant' – Which is right?* Available at www.unhcr.org/55df0e556.html. Accessed 18/01/16.

Weekers, J., Acuna, D.L., Sanchez, M.T. et al. (2009) *Developing a Public Health Workforce to Address Migrant Health Needs in Europe*. Brussels: International Organization for Migration.

World Health Organization (2010) *The WHO Global Code of Practice on the International Recruitment of Health Personnel*. Geneva: WHO.

World Health Organization (2014) *World Health Statistics 2014*. Geneva: WHO. [Online] Available at www.who.int/gho/publications/world_health_statistics/2014/en. Accessed 12/9/2016.

World Health Organization (2015) *Globalization*. [Online] Available at www.who.int/trade/glossary/story043/en. Accessed 30/08/15.

PART TWO

SKILLS, APPROACHES AND STYLES

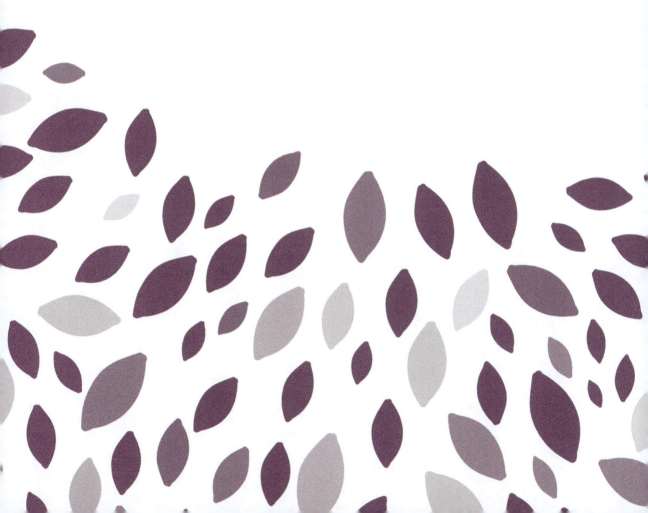

7 THE COACHING LEADER

Brian Webster-Henderson, Gillian McCready and Sandra Cairncross

---

Chapter learning outcomes

On completion of this chapter you will:

- Have a clear understanding of the concept of coaching from theoretical and practical perspectives.
- Have become familiar with the CLEAR coaching model and understand its various stages.
- Have knowledge of the applicability of coaching to your developing role as a nurse and how you might use coaching within a clinical learning environment.
- Have a rich understanding of the importance of the skills of listening and thinking, and how they can enhance your approach as a coaching leader in nursing.

Key concepts

Coaching, CLEAR model, listening, thinking, personal reflection

---

INTRODUCTION

This chapter takes a slightly different approach from others in this book, in that it presents to you an established approach – that of coaching – that is commonly used in other fields of work such as personal leadership development, mentoring and facilitation of thinking in organisations. The skills required in coaching and the frameworks that support it have a strong and connected value-set within the profession of nursing. Listening to patients, valuing others, giving patients, carers and colleagues undivided and focused attention in the way in which we relate to them, are values which are just as important in your everyday practice as a nurse as they are in the practice of coaching. To support your learning, this chapter focuses on providing you with an understanding of what coaching is, as well as introducing you to a framework to support your developing knowledge around coaching. We also introduce you to key skills and techniques that are important to develop your skillset in coaching, as well as providing you with some scenarios and activities to support your thinking. The skills used in coaching can be of value to you as a nurse in the way in which you interact with patients and relatives, as well as members of the nursing and inter-disciplinary professional teams found in a range of healthcare settings (Byrne, 2007). As such, coaching is as much about your own personal development as a professional, as it is about applying a skillset and way of interacting with others. At the heart of our thinking is the concept that nursing leadership requires individuals who are self-aware, reflective and actively demonstrate a skillset that others can look up to and admire alongside their professional integrity. As a student nurse, you are in the perfect position to hone these skills, and to use them as you develop personally and professionally in your own practice.

WHAT IS COACHING?

You will be familiar with coaching from sports – the football coach working with a team or the athletics coach working with a group of runners. You may be aware of the move towards coaches specialising in different areas, often focusing on specific areas of development. More recently coaching has moved into other areas: for example, lifestyle coaching and executive coaching have grown in popularity, with individuals seeking coaches to help them with a specific area for development such as support in managing work–life balance or in a transition to a leadership or management role. Coaching in all these contexts is essentially concerned with enhancing performance, often focusing on a particular area or goal. This view draws upon the work of Whitmore (2009: 10) who characterises coaching as:

> unlocking people's potential to maximise their own performance. It is helping them to learn rather than teaching them.

The way that we view coaching is as a combination of these: both as a means to assist people to find ways of doing things differently (whether that is a member of staff who wants to improve their performance in a particular skill, or a patient who wants to make some changes which aim to enhance their health), and as a means to assist with personal development more generally.

Many of you will also be familiar with mentoring – perhaps a more senior colleague mentoring a more junior one, or soon-to-be graduate nurses mentoring new student nurses. In your own experience you will have been used to working with mentors who undertake further training to learn how to support you as a student in the clinical practice learning environment. The terms coaching and mentoring are used interchangeably by some. Within this chapter we focus on coaching, which we believe to be different from mentoring. Coaching in this context focuses on a specific goal or area, as opposed to mentoring which can be seen as longer-term support in helping individuals to develop more generally.

Coaching provides a platform and interaction between individuals to understand a present situation, identify objectives, explore actions and review those actions to meet the desired outcomes. These elements are, of course, supported by a number of features or attributes including listening and questioning on the part of the coach. Listening and questioning aim to help the individual (patient/relative/team member) to explore the situation, and to enable them to self-identify the next steps that they need to take within their particular situation. The rationale behind this approach has parallels with more constructivist approaches to learning, in that knowledge is not something that can be transmitted but comes through engaging (Papert, 1990).

The benefits of a coaching approach are that it supports empowerment, self-awareness and a deeper insight that can be applied to a range of future situations by the individual. From a patient care perspective this is a fundamental attribute of nursing care. In addition, a coaching approach in nursing can increasingly be integrated into the workplace (Clutterbuck, 2003).

In relation to a coaching leadership approach when applied to colleague-to-colleague situations, it can be characterised as helping a colleague to solve a problem themselves, rather than solving it for them, or helping them to self-identify a solution rather than suggesting a solution to them. As you can imagine, this approach can (initially) take longer than suggesting a given way forward and indeed this is often cited as a barrier; a reason why a coaching approach can't be adopted. However, we would suggest that such a view is perhaps short-sighted in that by investing the time upfront, the nurse leader is helping to develop their colleague and enabling them to better solve problems on their own in future.

Becoming a coaching leader requires investment in skills to underpin this. The skills and techniques can be employed in different situations in the workplace to good effect. In particular, active listening and exploring options can be employed in meetings when discussing issues and can lead to the emergence of better solutions. The skills can also be used to 'manage upwards' (i.e. in working with a manager to understand what is expected in any given situation).

Activity 7.1

Take a moment to reflect on your reading of this chapter so far. Imagine that you have an interview for a new job and that one of the questions you are asked is:

> In hospital, we encourage all managers to adopt a coaching approach in their leadership.

- How would you describe what a coaching approach is?
- What benefits would coaching one of your team members bring you and them?
- How does a coaching approach already fit with your approach with patients?

What would you say?

Write your answers down – then read the section again and check your understanding.

THE CLEAR MODEL

This section of the chapter introduces you to a simple yet powerful coaching model. The CLEAR model aims to help you structure your conversations with team members and colleagues, and create an environment in which you can work collaboratively, respectfully and productively together. In addition, it aims to give you tools to enhance your interactions with patients. Professor Peter Hawkins and his colleagues developed the CLEAR model in the early 1980s (Hawkins and Smith, 2006). Figure 7.1 gives a summary of its stages.

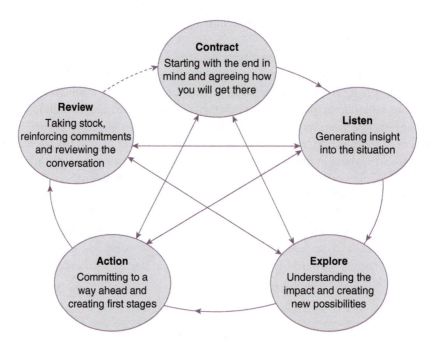

Figure 7.1 The CLEAR model

You will notice that there are arrows that connect the stages to each other, in a clockwise direction, and across the middle. CLEAR is not the linear process which may be suggested by the mnemonic, where you start at the beginning and step through each stage in turn. It is fluid and responsive – you can move back and forth between the stages in response to the needs and interests of the individual you are interacting with at that moment. The beauty of the CLEAR model over other coaching models is that it places an emphasis on *listening* and on the importance of *contracting* clearly ... but more of that later!

Activity 7.2

We are going to ask you to work with a partner throughout this chapter, to help you experience the benefits of adopting a coaching approach, and to practise the process and skills.

- Think about who you might like to work with for the remainder of your work through this chapter. You might, for example, approach a fellow student nurse on your programme who is also reading this book and set up a coaching partnership.
- Arrange to meet for an hour and a half to practise the CLEAR steps together.
- Now that you have arranged to meet, read the following sections that outline each of the stages in a CLEAR conversation. We have given you example questions that will help you understand the focus of each stage, and will give you prompts for your coaching conversation.

THE STAGES IN CLEAR

The stages in the CLEAR model are designed to provide a structured coaching approach. This chapter focuses now on the different aspects of the model and provides you with some example questions/approaches.

Contracting: Is about starting with the end in mind and agreeing how you will get there together.

Information box 7.1: Some useful questions to incorporate in your practice

What would you like to talk about today?

What do you want to achieve from our conversation?

What do you want to focus on in particular?

What would make our conversation successful?

How will we work together today?

How could I be most useful to you?

Before you start any meeting, project or working relationship, it is important to build a solid foundation by making sure that you understand each others' needs and expectations. Avoid the temptation to just get on with the work! When projects or relationships go wrong, it can often be traced back to a lack of open discussion and mutual understanding in their earliest stages.

Within nursing there are many examples where adopting this approach can be effective and can provide the patient or member of staff with a sense of confidence in the nurse and/or themselves, and can help them to feel valued – examples might include: when giving bad news; when spending time with a patient to discuss a particular issue; when meeting a client for the first time; when working with members of the nursing team.

Listen: Listening is a key component of the CLEAR model and is focused on generating insight into the situation. Listening is a skill that pays respectful attention to the details of the patient/client or staff member.

Information box 7.2: Examples of 'listening' questions/comments

Tell me more about ...

What more would you add?

How do other people see the situation?

What I have heard you say is ...

I am sensing that ...

The connections that I hear are ...

However, it is important when applying the skill of listening to be wary of becoming over-fascinated by the story. Your purpose in listening is not for you to understand the detail of the situation, but to enable the person you are interacting with to hear themselves and understand more about their own situation.

Explore: The explore stage of the CLEAR model is pivotal to its application. It allows you to understand the impact that the situation is having on the individual and helps you work with the individual to create new possibilities for action. In various nursing scenarios and when chosen appropriately this can facilitate a powerful nurse–patient or team interaction.

Information box 7.3: Examples of 'exploring' questions/comments

When you want to explore feelings:

How do you feel about that?

What assumptions might be getting in the way?

Reflecting back your observations:

    As you talk this through, what occurs to you?

    I notice that ...

Suggesting some options for the patient or team member to consider:

    Think of five things that you could do ...

    Who might help you with this?

It is important that you 'admire the problem' from every angle – that is, that you listen and think objectively with the individual at the centre of your attention and considerations. It is important to help the individual to be certain that the problem they said they wanted to solve is the right one. Having used this model in our own practice, a clear hint for good practice would be to consider if their 'presenting issue' is the one that needs to be addressed, or whether it is a symptom of a wider or deeper issue.

Action: Action is about committing to the way ahead and supporting the individual to create the next steps. In a patient-centred environment, or indeed an environment where care is pivotal to the culture, action is a vital step in completing the CLEAR model/process.

Information box 7.4: Examples of 'action' questions

    What are the pros and cons of each of your possible actions?

    What will you do to radically increase your chances of success?

    Who needs to be involved, consulted or informed?

    What is the first step that you will take?

    What will you say? Let's practise it now ...

    When precisely will you do that?

The individual's first step may seem small, but it is important to help the individual to be specific and confident about taking their first step as a way of facilitating their ability to move forward from the discussion or interaction you as a nurse are having with them.

Review: This final step in the CLEAR model is about taking stock, reinforcing commitments and reviewing the conversation. It is a vital completion to the process and key to ensuring that the previous steps of the interaction have addressed the individual's needs.

> ## Information box 7.5: Examples of 'review' questions
>
> What you will do next?
>
> What is clearer to you now?
>
> What have you learned?
>
> What feedback do we have for each other?
>
> When and how will we review your progress?

It is important when you apply the CLEAR model that as an individual you look back as well as forward, that you stand back from the detail and reflect. The CLEAR model is made up of five well-defined steps. Although its application to nursing may have been limited to date, we would suggest that it is an important contribution to patient-centred care. The introduction to this book described how some of the challenges of poor care were directly linked to poor nursing leadership in a range of reports. It is with this in mind that we would suggest the CLEAR model offers one framework in which you as a nurse can develop your skills of communication, listening and focused interaction in a planned and professional manner. Whilst it may seem 'odd' at first, the practice of focusing on individuals and creating a structured environment where you can listen and provide focused attention is key. Now take some time to practise what you have learned so far.

Activity 7.3 CLEAR practice session

To practise the CLEAR approach:

- Ask your partner to practise with you.
- Before meeting them, identify a challenge or an opportunity that you have ahead, and ask them to do the same. Your CLEAR conversation will give you protected time to think about it and work out what to do next.
- When you meet your partner, agree who will be the coach and who will be the coachee first, and set an alarm for half an hour.
- When the buzzer goes, swap roles and start the process again. You may like to set a warning sound for five minutes from the end of each of the half hour sessions.
- Follow the **CLEAR** process. Start with **Contracting** on how you will work together, move on to **Listening** to your partner's thinking, then move into the **Exploring**and **Action** stages to enable them to deepen their insight and identify first steps. Finish with a **Review**.

Remember that the most effective conversation will move fluidly between the stages of CLEAR, depending on the needs and interests of the coachee in that moment.

For example, you may need to move back to re-**Contract** on the coachee's desired outcomes for the conversation once they have explored their thinking in the **Listen** stage. Or, having moved on to agree **Actions**, the coachee may discover a block to progress that they need to think about further and so you will return to **Listen** for a while.

It is important for your learning that at the end of this practise session you both have time to do a **Review**. In discussing your experience of CLEAR, you may find it helpful to review and reflect on the following questions together:

- What did you find useful and rewarding about using the CLEAR process?
- What did you find unusual or difficult when using CLEAR?
- What will you do similarly next time, and what will you do differently?
- Crucially, what implications do the process and skills have for your leadership approach?

ADOPTING A COACHING APPROACH

As we hope you will have experienced, it is no coincidence that the model is called 'CLEAR'! You will have seen how it gives clarity to the stages in a coaching conversation, and how it brings about clarity of thought and action. A common concern about adopting a coaching approach is that it takes too much time. However, even the briefest conversation beside the coffee machine can be structured in this way, for example:

C: What would be useful right now?

L: Tell me the three most significant things about it.

E: How do you feel about it? What might you do?

A: What are you going to do and by when?

R: What are you taking away from this conversation?

With this in mind, we would suggest that the coaching conversation *can* be adopted into your everyday practice as a nurse: with a range of individuals that you may need to interact with. As a developing leader it allows you to develop your communication skills in a professional and structured manner. Once you are familiar with the CLEAR process, we suggest that you share it with the students with whom you work closely with on your programme, and possibly your mentors. Once they know that you will follow its steps in your discussions with them, whether in one-to-ones or in groups, they may be more prepared to either share their thinking or to help you differently as you look for ways to find solutions to issues and problems that you encounter in practice. When you are a qualified nurse and are leading a team, by adopting a coaching approach, you will show your team members that you believe in their capacity to develop, to think independently and creatively, and to take personal responsibility for their work. The more involved your team members are, the more motivated, independent and skilled they will be. And that can only lead to better performance and productivity, to everyone's benefit!

LISTENING INTENTLY, THINKING DEEPLY

It is vital that the skills of listening and thinking are practised to a high standard within a coaching approach. One of the greatest gifts that we can give to a colleague or friend is to be there for them, to give them time to think and be truly heard, by themselves as well as by you. When we hear ourselves think out loud, we discover things that we have not yet brought to conscious awareness, and see connections and possibilities that we had not realised were there. It would be easy for us to write 'to *simply* be there', but it is not simple or easy to be truly present, fully attentive, and to listen – really listen. It takes skill, focus and will.

Imagine what would happen if you were to poke a stick between someone's bicycle spokes as they were riding along. It would stop them in their tracks, with painful consequences. Interrupting has the same impact. As Nancy Kline (2010) said, 'When we come in too soon, we can extinguish fresh, even brilliant, independent thinking'.

Activity 7.4

We call this activity 'Two Deadly Sins'. What you need to do is hum a favourite tune. While you are humming it, try to recall the theme tune for the television programme that you watched last night.

Impossible, right?! Listening to someone talk about an issue while you are thinking about the advice you wish to offer is like trying to recall a tune while another tune is playing. It is a remarkable thought, but you can help your coachee to achieve more by appearing to do nothing. Give yourself permission to do less, not more. Know that your fully attentive presence is a catalyst for their thinking, and watch and enjoy the results. However, simple can be mistaken for easy. Really attentive, focused listening, without interrupting or giving in to the temptation to give advice, is hard … but brilliantly effective. As you develop the skills of listening and thinking you should take time to rehearse with a trusted colleague or peer.

Activity 7.5

Arrange to meet the partner that you practised the CLEAR model with and this time focus on listening. Try this 'Thinking Pair' exercise, which is based on Nancy Kline's approach to a thinking partnership (Kline, 1999: 142–7).

- Agree to give each other five uninterrupted minutes of thinking out loud time.
- Set the timer and ask your partner: 'What would you like to think about and what are your thoughts?
- Settle back and listen. Look directly at your partner. Think only about what they are saying, knowing that the more present you are, the deeper and more productive their thinking will be.
- They may pause, but don't be tempted to jump in. They may still be thinking, silently.
- When they have finished their 'wave of thinking', they will say so in some way. 'That's me.' 'I'm done.' 'I can't think of anything else.' But they will!
- Ask: 'What *more* do you think, or feel, or want to say?'
- And you will find that they do indeed have more to say, to think about, to discover, to decide. You can ask the same question several times and each time a new thought will come to mind.
- When the timer goes, swap roles.

This activity is a really effective way of developing your skills of undivided listening. It is often an idea at the end of this activity to create an opportunity where you both tell each other what you appreciate about each other: not about what they did, but about a quality in them, for example, 'I appreciate your ability to challenge yourself', 'I appreciate the clarity of your thinking', 'I appreciate your support'. Giving appreciation is a strong skill as well as a delight.

As with activity 7.3, you may also find it helpful to take the time to review the Thinking Pair exercise and the following questions may support you in doing that:

What did you think and how did you feel about your Thinking Pair?

How will you introduce Thinking Pairs to your team, now or in the future?

How will you continue thinking together? Weekly is good!

Thinking, listening and appreciating in Thinking Pairs takes practice. With more experience, you will be able to increase the time that you give to each other to 10 minutes or even more. You will notice that you become more and more hungry for uninterrupted thinking time, and that your Thinking Pairs become a vital part of your leadership toolkit. It is important that as you develop this skill with a colleague or peer that you can also apply it to your interaction with patients. Providing a patient in your care with uninterrupted time is a quality of interaction that is key to that patient's experience of care.

LISTENING IN CLEAR

The CLEAR process integrates both listening and making observations in the **Listen** stage. First, it encourages you to allow your coachee to speak about their issue without any interruption or intervention, other than saying things such as, 'Tell me more about …' and 'What more would you add?' (the Thinking Pair questions, while slightly different, achieve the same end). Over time, this approach will encourage your coachee to use this time not to paint the picture for you, but for themselves. You will find, in fact, that if they know you value their thinking, and you believe that they may well have the answers, they will use the time to solve the issue themselves. How great is that as a leader, not having to do all the thinking?! You will also notice that they will tend to talk about whatever they need and want to say early in your meetings, irrespective of any questions that you ask or the observations that you make. It is only later, when they feel heard, that they will be able to respond to what you might say. It is only once they have 'told their story' that they can move on to consider your insights or challenges.

NEVER UNDERESTIMATE THE IMPORTANCE OF LISTENING

You may feel that in order to be an effective, respected, leader that you have to have all the answers; that your team member or patient will expect you to have them; that you won't be earning your title (or your salary) if you don't. You may not have all the answers, but now you do know the right questions to ask! What a release and an opportunity. By looking at things in this way, you are giving yourself permission *not* to know, and showing that you understand that one of your most important functions is to enable others to think, and to know differently from you. We don't need to be an expert in all aspects of our function, but we do need to become an expert in knowing when to direct, and when to facilitate – to know when to tell and when to let someone work something out for themselves. Listening, really listening, being there and being present can also increase your presence and help in making connections (Su and Wilkins, 2013).

Maybe you have knowledge or expertise that your team member doesn't, or maybe you are in a crisis or against a tight deadline. Maybe there is only one correct way to do something (and not just the way you like it to be done). That is when to be directive, to tell or instruct. However, if you want to enable your colleague, team member or patient to learn, to be creative, or you understand they have the answer but just don't know it yet, be non-directive. Facilitate their thinking by helping them tap into their experience and expertise, and identify the answer for themselves. Often, coaching is thought to be a wholly non-directive process. In fact, the best leader knows how to flex throughout the spectrum and use all of its skills. See Figure 7.2, which offers an overview of coaching: the 'coaching spectrum' (Downey, 2003). As the title suggests, it provides a summary of the approaches used across the directive (approaches that you would use to solve someone else's problem *for* them) and non-directive spectrum (where you would help the individual to identify their own solutions and solve the problem themselves).

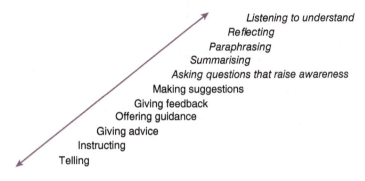

Non-directive
Helping someone solve their own problem

Listening to understand
Reflecting
Paraphrasing
Summarising
Asking questions that raise awareness
Making suggestions
Giving feedback
Offering guidance
Giving advice
Instructing
Telling

Directive
Solving someone's problem for them

Figure 7.2 The coaching spectrum

Activity 7.6

We call this activity 'Match and Mismatch'.

Think about a time recently when you were told what to do and how to do it, and reflect on how you felt. Were you pleased? Or were you annoyed? Did you want to resist the instructions or follow them?

Now think about a time when someone didn't tell you what to do, but asked you questions to get you to think about the answer or to work out how to do it for yourself. Did you feel supported and enabled, or did you feel anxious and confused?

If you had one or more of the negative reactions above, the chances are that the person misunderstood your current knowledge or skill in this particular area and so mismatched their approach to your need. If on the other hand you felt positive about their interventions, this would suggest that they matched the level of direction you needed and gave you what was useful. Wittingly or unwittingly, they matched their approach to your need.

You may find Table 7.1 (the 'coaching continuum', Downey, 2003) helpful. It highlights actions and behaviours from the coach (in this case you) against directive and non-directive behaviours and skills.

One of the most important aspects of becoming an effective coaching leader is identifying what a patient's or team member's needs are in a particular moment. You may find that within one conversation, they would value your guidance on one thing, and would like to think for themselves about another. For example, a patient may know the kind of diet that they need to eat in order to ensure they are as healthy as they can be.

Table 7.1   The coaching continuum

Coachee's needs	Knowledge and skills	Skills and confidence	Independent problem solving	Ongoing learning and continuous improvement
Coachee's behaviour	Enthusiastic and interested	Confused or frustrated	Self critical, hesitant or bored	Confident
	Lacks knowledge, skills and experience	Has some knowledge, skills and experience	Is capable	Is fully competent
	Is willing to be led	Has variable commitment	Is often self-directed	Is self-reliant
Coaching focus	Skills coaching	Performance coaching	Development coaching	Transformation coaching
Coaching technique	Instructing	Involving	Facilitating	Empowering
Coach's actions	Listen and ask	Listen and ask	Listen and ask	Listen and ask
	Tell, explain and check	Explain, involve and encourage	Support and collaborate	Affirm and challenge
	Give and ask for feedback	Give and ask for feedback	Give and ask for feedback	Give and ask for feedback

On the other hand, they may not know how best to exercise to achieve the best results for their particular situation. So, if you were to tell the patient about relevant exercise, they might feel relieved and motivated. But if you were to tell them what to eat, they might feel irritated or patronised. In addition, it would waste their time and might diminish their commitment to further learning in that context. Even within one task, you may need to adopt different approaches, depending on the skills and experiences of the individual you are interacting with. Sometimes, it can be hard to work out what is needed, and when, so you can take the pressure off yourself and ask! As part of the **Contracting** stage, and throughout your conversation, you can ask the individual you are interacting with what would help them most. Be attuned to their behaviour and reactions to your approach. If you sense resistance or anxiety, ask them how they are feeling, what is getting in the way and what they need from you in order to feel more confident and committed in that moment. But of course, if you were to be the individual's manager, you carry the ultimate responsibility for the work they do and its success. So, if you think that their decisions and actions would benefit from your input, or you need something done in a particular way, it is appropriate and necessary for you to give direction and be directive. A truly effective leader flexes up and down the coaching spectrum as the situation and the individual's knowledge and skills demand.

Coaching is not a new approach in nursing; there is evidence within the literature of its use in a range of settings and of various coaching approaches (Collins and Fillery-Travis, 2015; Mitchell et al., 2013; Williamson, 2009). Within this chapter we have focused on an approach to coaching that values the skills of listening and thinking and how to use these skills in a meaningful, respectful and professional way and have suggested the use of the CLEAR model. Listening is not a new skill but an important and pivotal part of excellent patient care (Wright, 2006). It is within this context of high quality patient care that the coaching approach here is positioned.

SUMMARY

Some key points from this chapter are:

- The skills of listening, reflecting and thinking are compatible with excellent nursing care.
- The use of a structured coaching model (in this case CLEAR) provides a focus for interactions with patients, staff and others.
- Not to over-emphasise the point, but *listening* is absolutely crucial in coaching, and a skill that requires practice.

FURTHER RESOURCES

Kline, N. (2009) *More Time to Think*. Leeds: Fisher King Publishing.
This book provides a further expansion from her original *Time to Think* book and is a useful source for developing your skills.

To access further resources related to this chapter, please visit the companion website at https://study.sagepub.com/taylor

REFERENCES

Byrne, G. (2007) 'Guest Editorial: Unlocking the potential – coaching as a means to enhance leadership and role performance in nursing'. *Journal of Clinical Nursing*, 16(11): 1987–8.
Clutterbuck, D. (2003) *Creating a Coaching Climate*. London: Clutterbuck Associates.
Collins, R. and Fillery-Travis, A. (2015) 'Transdisciplinary problems: the teams addressing them and their support through team coaching'. Chapter 3 in Gibbs, P. (Ed.) *Transdisciplinary Professional Learning and Practice*. Switzerland: Springer.
Downey, M. (2003) *Effective Coaching: Lessons from the Coach's Coach*. Florence, KY: Texere Publishing.
Hawkins, P. and Smith, N. (2006) *Coaching, Mentoring and Organisational Consultancy*. Berkshire: Open University Press, McGraw-Hill.
Kline, N. (1999) *Time to Think*. London: Cassell Illustrated.
Kline, N. (2010) *What Happens in the Silence? The Real Art of Coaching*. [Online] Available at www.timetothink.com/uploaded/BACP%20Speech%2017%20Ju.
Mitchell, G.J., Cross, N., Wilson, M., Biernacki, S., Wong, W., Adib, B. and Rush, D. (2013) 'Complexity and health coaching: synergies in nursing'. *Nursing Research and Practice Annual*, 2013 (Article ID 238620): 1–7.

Papert, S. (1990) 'An introduction to the 5th Anniversary collection'. In Harel, I. (Ed.) *Constructionist Learning: A 5th Anniversary Collection of Papers.* Cambridge, MA: MIT Media Laboratory.

Su, A.J. and Wilkins, M.M. (2013) *Own the Room.* Boston: Harvard Business Review Press

Whitmore, J. (2009) *Coaching for Performance: Growing Human Potential and Purpose – The Principles and Practice of Coaching and Leadership*, 4th edition. London: Nicholas Brealey Publishing.

Williamson, C. (2009) 'Using life coaching techniques to enhance leadership skills in nursing'. *Nursing Times*, 105(8): 20–3.

Wright, S. (2006) 'The beauty of silence: deep listening is a key nursing skill that can be learned'. *Nursing Standard*, 20(50): 18–20.

8 NETWORKING AND LEADERSHIP

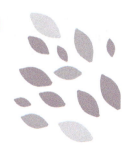

Ruth Taylor and Susan Tokley

Chapter learning outcomes

On completion of this chapter you will be able to:

- Describe theories of networking in the context of leadership.
- Apply theories of networking to the practice of healthcare leadership.
- Evaluate the use of social media for networking in the context of professional practice.
- Map your own networks and collate a set of tools to develop your networks for your own leadership practice.

Key concepts

Networks, social media, mapping of networks, professional issues

---

INTRODUCTION

The purpose of this chapter is to offer an overview of the theories of networking and their application or links to healthcare (nursing) practice. We think this is a growing area of importance for all leaders – whether they are experienced practitioners or, like you, students who are developing their professional practice and understanding.

We start this chapter by laying out some of the theory and then move on to consider that theory in relation to your own and others' practice. The activities that we use aim to get you to think about the importance of networking – what it can bring to both professional practice and to your own professional development. The activities will also give you the opportunity to try out new ways of networking, or to build on what you already do. A key focus is on social media – this is a growing area for professional networking.

You may already use a variety of social media tools in your personal life. This will give you a head start in being able to navigate the social media world as a professional. Whilst we advocate the use of social media for networking, we will also focus in on the associated professional issues so that you can confidently use the tools without fear of inappropriate professional behaviour.

THEORIES OF NETWORKING IN THE CONTEXT OF LEADERSHIP

What are the theories of networking in the context of leadership? Social scientists have recently developed something called 'network theory' as a new way of understanding the world (Baines and Hale, 2004). At a basic level a network is a system or circuit that allows information, ideas or favours to flow. You may find out about something new through this route rather than via advertising, for example. This theoretical approach tries to set out how things or people link with each other in order to develop. When the framework is applied to people it is often referred to as 'social network theory': a set of people or a group with a pattern of interactions or ties between them. Networking is essential for professions such as nursing where communication between people is important as a means to the delivery of key activities related to care or treatment. In addition, according to network theory, personal success is directly linked to the networks you join. It is therefore important to understand and consider networking in relation to the development of your leadership and clinical skills and knowledge, so that you can continually improve patient care, and for the development of your career.

Networking involves creating or finding a support system of individuals or groups with the same or similar interests and objectives, and with internal or external links to yourself or your organisation so that these networks can be developed and used. Most simply it is about establishing helpful relationships with people who will support you to move forward with whatever your issue is. For example, it could be to help with accessing extra resources or for learning and gaining knowledge and expertise, or to find opportunities for career progression.

Duncan Watts (2004), Associate Professor of Sociology at Columbia University, New York, considers that the majority of people can be linked to each other by six steps: 'six degrees of separation'. This theory suggests that we probably already know people with the links to those other people who can help us get the personal contacts that we need for our professional networking. So all you need to do is work out who could help you and make contact!

So how does networking fit with leadership? As a clinician, at whatever level, even when starting out in your career, you will need to demonstrate and provide leadership in your clinical practice on behalf of patients or colleagues in a variety of situations. This leadership may involve managing individual patient care needs as a student under supervision, or working as part of a team to manage the delivery of care for a group of patients, or speaking up about unsafe care or practice. The Nursing and Midwifery

Council Code (NMC, 2015) has a number of statements within it that can be linked to the need to network to ensure you meet professional standards of practice (see information box 8.1).

Information box 8.1: The NMC Code and networking

Practise effectively:

8. Work cooperatively

To achieve this, you must:

8.2 maintain effective communication with colleagues

8.6 share information to identify and reduce risk

9. Share your skills, knowledge and experience for the benefit of people receiving care and your colleagues

To achieve this, you must:

9.2 gather and reflect on feedback from a variety of sources, using it to improve your practice and performance

9.4 support students' and colleagues' learning to help them develop their professional competence and confidence

Promote professionalism and trust:

20. Uphold the reputation of your profession at all times

20.1 keep to and uphold the standards and values set out in the Code

20.7 make sure you do not express your personal beliefs (including political, religious or moral beliefs) to people in an inappropriate way

20.8 act as a role model of professional behaviour for students and newly qualified nurses and midwives to aspire to

Whilst reading the Code statements in information box 8.1, you may have thought about the need for you to network with colleagues and mentors in a reciprocal way as an approach to improving your own and others' practice. You may also have thought about the need for you to be a model of integrity and leadership for others to aspire to, and this is relevant in networking as you will be seen and heard by all sorts of other people as you grow your connections.

Grossman and Valiga (2013) believe that networks are vital for providing access to contacts, referrals, information, support, feedback, understanding and empathy for developing leaders. They see intra-professional and inter-professional collaboration and networking as key and as the means for nurses to maintain professional identity as well as a route to working toward organisational, professional or societal reform. To apply their thinking to your role as a student nurse, their stance is that to grow as a person and as a professional and leader you should develop your professional networks internally and externally to your organisation and then use them. Griffey (2009) sees networking as a skill for leaders linked to the ability to adapt to new initiatives. As you become more senior, networks will expand and may include politicians, universities, and executive colleagues, service users, and other influential groups and individuals.

Individuals can feel empowered by having the opportunity to network and the subsequent informal power gained by developing networks of alliances with peers (Enterkin et al., 2013). Positive relationships can be demonstrated between empowerment, job satisfaction and intention to remain in post or the nursing profession, thus showing what an essential support mechanism networking is to prevent isolation and in overall development as a leader.

Marshall (2011) looked at a number of theories and models related to nurse leadership and management. Transformational leadership that effects change and 'nurse leadership knowing' (i.e. passing on the knowledge of how to nurse at all levels) are popular concepts within complex Western healthcare systems. However, for the future she predicts that the challenge will be for nursing to create better evidence for best practice in clinical leadership. Inter-professional engagement in the bigger picture of healthcare will be essential, and so networking with other healthcare professionals will be key for the future of leadership development in healthcare and in creating this evidence-base. She sees people skills (which include networking and working collaboratively) as part of the important attributes for nursing leaders which would allow nursing to drive this forward. These attributes were identified by Carroll (2005) and are listed in information box 8.2.

Information box 8.2: Important attributes for nurse leaders

- Personal integrity.
- Strategic vision.
- Action orientation.
- Team building.
- Communication.
- Management.
- Technical competence.
- *People skills.*
- Personal survival skills/attributes.

It's possible to make a case that these attributes are *all* relevant to networking. Communities of practice are seen as key to the development of situations in which individuals are able to influence and effect change (Marshall, 2011). The world does not change one person at a time: it changes as people form networks around common causes. Communities of practice evolve from networks, which multiply to allow new systems to emerge that eventually create change. The ability to see emerging trends on the horizon and tap into them as a leader will come from being part of networks. Sharing and discussing ideas with like-minded individuals to influence and determine the direction of change enables supportive and collaborative approaches to be a part of your community of practice.

Eventually you will find that you will want to expand your networks so as to embrace others outside your immediate profession and even outside healthcare as a way of informing your views and developing your thinking. Making contact with new groups and individuals will generate energy and create ideas and make your work more fulfilling and productive.

Activity 8.1

Draw a 'mindmap' or make a list of your current connections and networks. Remember to include people and organisations that sit outside of healthcare. Note the purpose of the connection (is it for professional information, support, learning, etc.?), and then think about whether there are any 'gaps' in your networks that you'd like to think of filling.

Think about all the things you have done and the people you will have met:

- School.
- Jobs.
- University or college.
- Courses or evening classes.
- Friends and family.
- Other acquaintances.
- Events and conferences you have attended.
- Placements, colleagues, mentors.
- Social media, LinkedIn, Facebook, etc.

Undertaking this activity may have given you confidence that you are already well-connected. At the same time, you may have identified some areas where you could do with further support. This is all good. Now you can start to think about how you engage with others to grow those connections. You can now see how powerful and important the need to network is and how it fits so closely with so many elements of successful leadership.

NETWORKING AND HEALTHCARE PRACTICE

Nurses, who are at the frontline of healthcare, collaborate with a whole range of individuals and organisations within their professional roles: with patients and their families, other nursing staff, medical staff and other health professionals, academics, students, the community and the general public, statutory organisations and government, and others (Ressler and Glazer, 2010). We have already alluded to some of the benefits of networking and this short section aims simply to clarify those benefits so that you can really think about how networking can help your own healthcare practice. Networking can link you to individuals, groups and organisations within and across your own area of practice so that you can:

- Deliver better care.
- Ensure that the right person/role holder is providing relevant input into a particular healthcare situation.
- Identify the most appropriate treatment or intervention.
- Discuss appropriate treatments or interventions with experts.
- Get access to relevant resources to enhance healthcare practice.
- Pick up the phone and quickly make contact with people who can help you.
- Offer advice or other input to others who need help.
- Gain support for your own practice, particularly in relation to managing your own emotional reactions to challenging healthcare or practice situations.
- Advocate for better healthcare practice (e.g. access to healthcare resources).
- Put patients and others in touch with organisations or people who can provide relevant support.
- Influence health policy and practice by being 'in on' the right conversations.

We are sure that you can think of more examples!

SOCIAL MEDIA AND NETWORKING

Networking, these days, does not have to be face-to-face. Social media (SoMe) can play an important role in all areas of networking, and in particular in relation to engagement with health and social care policy – as you will see as we share examples of useful SoMe sites in this section of our chapter. Having made this positive statement, it is worth saying that SoMe is relatively untested in terms of its evidence-base as a vehicle for good within healthcare practice, and at times its use seems to be accepted uncritically as good. Many commentators are, though, convincing in their descriptions of the value of SoMe, citing the way that it can drive social change, and lead to meaningful engagement across and within communities (Ferguson, 2013). We subscribe to this perspective.

It is probable (though not certain of course) that you are already an active virtual networker – you may be networking 'on the go' with your portable devices. Do you have a Twitter, Facebook, LinkedIn or Instagram account for example? How many 'friends' or 'followers' do you have, and are any of these people that you have never actually met in 'real' life? (Philosophical question … What *is* real life?) You may use one or more SoMe sites for professional purposes, or, at the moment, use them purely for social purposes. What we aim to convince you of (if you need convincing!) is that SoMe is an excellent way to create networks for professional purposes. We should embrace SoMe (Barry and Hardiker, 2012) in a world where nursing practice is beginning to be influenced by the discussions that go on, and the connections that are created in this space. Although Schmitt et al. (2012) assert that nurses are generally late adopters of technology (possibly due to age-related factors), our own experiences of SoMe and nursing are that many nurses are at the forefront of its use for professional practice and have led the way.

What do we mean by the term 'social media'? It is defined as:

> the constellation of Internet-based tools that help a user to connect, collaborate, and communicate with others in real time. Social media enables one to participate in active, digital dialog or conversation in contrast to a passive, digital monologue, for example, the reading of a static webpage. (Ressler and Glazer, 2010: 1)

Kaplan and Haenlein (2010: 61) describe the six main types of SoMe as follows:

- Collaborative products (e.g. Wikipedia).
- Blogs and microblogs (e.g. Twitter).
- Content communities (e.g. YouTube).
- Social networking sites (e.g. Facebook).
- Virtual game worlds (e.g. World of Warcraft).
- Virtual social worlds (e.g. Second Life).

More specifically, Koteyko et al. (2015: 468) define social networking sites as 'a tool, a conduit for information and a traversable space'. They are 'web-based services that allow users to create public profiles, pages and groups, articulate connections to other users'. For the purposes of this chapter, the ones that we are most interested in are blogs and microblogs, and social networking sites. However, this does not mean that the other SoMe forms do not hold the potential for networking opportunities.

PROFESSIONAL CONSIDERATIONS

It is important to note that whilst we strongly advocate the use of SoMe as a form of professional networking and engagement, there can of course be some aspects to SoMe that need consideration from a professional perspective. Piscotty et al. (2015) have identified some of the benefits and risks of SoMe within nursing. Whilst they identify the potential value of SoMe aiding nurse communication with patients and families, they also highlight the risks of nurses using SoMe inappropriately or unprofessionally, and urge nurses to think carefully about what they post on SoMe from a professional perspective. Equally some other authors have focused on the personal use of SoMe and electronic devices by healthcare workers whilst giving nursing care, and their potential to lead to errors of care (Brady et al., 2009; Kalisch and Aebersold, 2010). Overall we would encourage you to engage with SoMe but be mindful of your own professional responsibilities in how you engage.

So, what can SoMe do for you in your professional practice and how do these things relate to the topic of this chapter? There are many ways, all of which derive from the concept of networking – whether it is simply about receiving information, or whether it is broader and leads to the development of connections with other people that have an impact on your professional practice. One of the authors has written elsewhere about the concept of social capital and networking (Taylor, 2013). This theoretical perspective enables us to see networking in light of the opportunities that it brings to create social capital. Briefly, social capital is a concept that is defined variously but probably most famously by Putnam (1995: 65) as:

> The features of social organizations such as networks, norms and social trust that facilitate coordination and co-operation for mutual benefit.

More simply put, social capital is encapsulated by Field's (2008) phrase, 'relationships matter'. For those of you who are interested, both these references provide a good overview of social capital theory, but for the purposes of this chapter, the idea is that the development of social capital is key to creating connections across individuals and organisations. The benefits of the development of social capital include: sharing of best practice, the development of good ideas and their subsequent enaction, provision of support to help with resilience, access to resources and knowledge that might not otherwise be available, and the ability to work towards common goals within a climate of supportive challenge. As you will see, SoMe seems to be a way through which many of these benefits can be realised. To illustrate this point, information box 8.3 provides a summary of the ways in which engagement with SoMe can be helpful. To balance the discussion, some of the disadvantages or concerns with SoMe are cited in information box 8.4.

Information box 8.3: Uses for social media

(Adapted from: Barry and Hardiker, 2012; Ressler and Glazer, 2010; Schmitt et al., 2012; Lawson and Cowling, 2014.)

- Improving health, for example through the awareness of health issues.
- Access to resources and information for healthcare.
- Communication and networking.
- Transcending communications across geographical and professional boundaries.
- Creating greater understanding of a whole range of issues for students, and can be used as a teaching medium, for example:

  o Communication skills.
  o Health policy.

    o   Patient privacy and ethics.
    o   Writing competencies.

- Offering opportunities to influence, for example on particular policy decisions.
- Understanding others' experiences, for example Dr Kate Granger's experience of having cancer (see Twitter @GrangerKate).

Information box 8.4: Possible risks in the use of social media

(Adapted from: Barry and Hardiker, 2012; Ressler and Glazer, 2010; Ferguson, 2013.)

- Unmoderated content, therefore it may be difficult to know if the content is evidence-based and robust.
- Issues with privacy.
- Publicly available in perpetuity (even if 'deleted').
- Possible professional concerns, for example:

    o   Confidentiality.
    o   Inappropriate sharing of information.
    o   Personal boundary issues.

- Workforce knowledge deficits so that it is not used to its full potential.
- Possible organisational risk, for example reduced productivity at work.
- A lack of evidence to support or refute its use for learning.

Activity 8.2 aims to help you to think about how SoMe is, or could be, part of your way of networking and communication more generally.

Activity 8.2

Do you think that SoMe is revolutionising the way that you communicate? Or is it something that you feel has always been part of your life? As a start, list the SoMe sites that you engage with and identify what, if any, professional activity you take part in in that context. Then have a look around these SoMe sites and come up with a list of possible ways of interacting professionally in this space.

If you think about the 'spread' of SoMe on a global basis, you can probably see that in your own existing networks you have 'friends' or 'followers' who span the globe. By the time you read this book, it is almost certain that the statistics will demonstrate an even wider spread than currently. Information box 8.5 offers an overview of the key statistics that demonstrate just how widely SoMe is used.

Information box 8.5: The 'spread' of social media – the number of users

Worldwide: 3,270,490,584 (45% of the population).

Africa: 313,257,074 (27% of the population).

Asia: 1,563,208,143 (38.8% of the population).

Europe: 604,122,380 (73.5% of the population).

Middle East: 115,823,882 (49% of the population).

North America: 313,862,863 (87.9% of the population).

Latin America/Caribbean: 333,115,908 (53.9% of the population).

Oceania/Australia: 27,100,334 (72.9% of the population).

(internetworldstats.com, as at 30/06/15)

From this we can see that SoMe is a global phenomenon – one which is certainly changing lives in small ways every day. We would assert that SoMe has the potential to change lives in big ways, and there are examples of where this has happened. Do you remember the 2011 riots in London that followed the death of Mark Duggan? He was shot dead by police in August of that year. The organisation of those riots was partly due to the use of SoMe. In addition, it is an example of how SoMe can not only exert some control over events, but can also be used to record events as they happen. This event is not healthcare related, but does provide an example of the power of SoMe on a national stage. Care crosses professional and organisational boundaries (some of these are global), and we therefore need 'cross cutting ties', Scott and Hofmeyer (2007: 4) that bring people and ideas together. We go on to discuss the example of the '6Cs' further on in the chapter – illustrating how SoMe can cut across those boundaries, bring people together, and develop an idea into something that has become somewhat of a national phenomenon.

Activity 8.3

If you don't already have a Twitter account, set one up. It is easy! Go to the website (http://twitter.com). Make sure that you choose a Twitter 'handle' (name) that is professional, and write a short biography that clearly demonstrates you are interested in professional issues. We suggest that you do the following:

- Follow a number (maybe 40) of profession-related Twitter users (information box 8.7 has some suggestions).
- Start commenting on people's postings – perhaps choose a topic area that you are interested in.

- Select a # conversation (hashtags enable users of Twitter to engage in conversation with others who are interested in similar areas of practice) about healthcare practice that is going on and read through the comments. Post a few comments of your own that demonstrate reflective skills, critical analysis skills, and a willingness to engage in open debate and discussion.
- We have setup a # for our book (#StudentNurseLeaders). We will use this as a way to connect with the readers of our book, and you will be able to share thoughts and resources with each other. We'd be delighted if you place a comment and join the conversation!

You might like to think about the kinds of national and international audiences that engage with SoMe and the impact that they are having, or could have, in your area of professional practice. Information box 8.6 lists some organisations that use SoMe to converse with the world, whether through information-giving, education, debate or challenge.

Information box 8.6: Organisations on Twitter

World Health Organization: @WHO

Royal College of Nursing: @theRCN

Nursing and Midwifery Council: @nmcnews

Scottish Government: @scotgov

Department of Health: @DHgovuk

Florence Nightingale Foundation: @FNightingaleF

In the world of healthcare, including in nursing and midwifery which seem to be big players in social media, SoMe is being used to transform who we have conversations with, and how we have those conversations. The potential for you as an individual to have an impact through SoMe seems much greater than through 'traditional' networking approaches which rely on you being in the right place at the right time. Think about England's '6Cs' (described below) – do you think it would have caught on without SoMe?

Jane Cummings (the Chief Nursing Officer for England) developed a three year strategy for nursing, midwifery and care staff – Compassion in Practice – which was launched in 2012. Within it, she identified the 6Cs (care, compassion, competence, communication, courage and commitment). Many of you will be familiar with these as they are becoming embedded within pre-registration nursing courses in England. SoMe was used to create conversations, send out messages, and embed some of the ideas within the zeitgeist. Some of us may query whether this is an example of where SoMe was used cleverly to capture the imagination of the professions leading to the spread of an idea that, in fact, was based on little evidence. That is not to say that the 6Cs in themselves are inappropriate values to aspire to – just that SoMe provided a vehicle for something that possibly should have taken longer to develop through the use of evidence and stronger consultation. What do you think? How about our own 6Cs for SoMe networking?

Connectivity
Communication
Collaboration
Curiosity
Co-operation
Collegiality

Information box 8.7 offers suggestions of Twitter users who you may wish to follow.

Information box 8.7: Suggestions of people and organisations to follow on Twitter

@ruthft1 (Ruth Taylor, book editor).

@bjw46 (Brian Webster-Henderson, book editor).

@WeNurses (connecting nurses to share information, ideas and knowledge).

@NurChat (fortnightly nurse tweet chats).

@jadvnursing (*Journal of Advanced Nursing*).

@BJNursing (*British Journal of Nursing*).

@TheKingsFund (independent charity working to improve health and healthcare in England).

We end this section with words of encouragement – encouragement to use the tools that are literally at your fingertips to develop your networks so that you can do more of all the things that we have described in this chapter. Not only will you benefit from growing your connections, but others will benefit from having you as part of their network too!

MAPPING YOUR NETWORKS

So how do you work out what your networks are and expand them? Some people are natural networkers. These people are described as connectors by Malcolm Gladwell in his book *The Tipping Point* (2002). Connectors seem to have the ability to see links and synergies between people and therefore bring those people together. They appear to like other people in a genuine and powerful way. To develop attributes of being more like a connector you may need to cultivate curiosity and an interest in people in a genuine away, avoiding being judgemental and seeing everyone as a possible member of a web of connections. The concept of social intelligence and the importance of developing and honing the ability to empathise and relate to others is described as the ability to get along well with others and to facilitate co-operation with you (Albrecht, 2006). Authenticity and empathy are especially important in social networking and it is better to have strong, authentic relationships with a manageable number of key people rather than trying to network with as many people as possible (Buggy, 2006). Buggy explores the pre-requisites for successful career networking – reflecting some of the social capital theory that we have discussed including the need to build trust, be authentic and take time to develop relationships.

If you are an introvert by nature, you can still build close co-operative relationships with a few people who are super networkers and gain benefits as if you were one of those super networkers (do you think you know any, or are you one yourself?). Having a few good colleagues who love to network and can link you into those networks can facilitate the development of your connections. In other words, if you're not super outgoing, you can take time, get comfortable, and build lasting supportive networks in ways that suit your own personality.

Go back to activity 8.1 and think about your current networks and your initial thoughts about 'gaps' in your networks. Now do activity 8.4.

Activity 8.4

What sorts of networks do you or will you need?

- Formal or informal?
- Personal.
- Professional.
- Clinical.
- Strategic clinical.
- Research.

What approaches can you take to developing your networks? Here are some examples for you to consider. Perhaps note down some ideas of how you will progress one or more of these.

- Join an existing professional network.
- Consider the SoMe options.
- Talk to your colleagues and seek introductions.
- Attend a professional event (take business cards or your contact details so you can stay in touch).

Most of what we have been saying has focused on the positive aspects of networking, but we do know that for some people networking can be a challenge. What are the blocks to networking? At this stage you might want to reflect on the things that are stopping you (if anything is stopping you!). Take five minutes out to jot down any concerns you might have.

Activity 8.5

What is stopping you from developing your networks? What can you do to move past those blockers?

We have come up with a list of possible blockers (and some suggestions to unblock them).

- Can't see the point.

  If there isn't a point, don't do it. Otherwise focus on the 'big picture' of growing your network for reasons that will motivate you – for example, career development, improvements in patient care.

- Managed fine so far without networking.

  You probably have, but think about whether there are gaps in your knowledge, skills, support systems that could benefit from input from others.

- Not confident in talking to strangers.

  This can be challenging for some people, but remember that even those who seem most confident may not be; and take small steps by setting a goal of talking to one new person at an event coffee break and exchanging contact details.

- Who would be interested in me? Don't like selling myself.

  The simple answer to that is – lots of people will be interested in you! But it's sometimes hard to feel that isn't it? Attend an event in an area of your expertise and make a point of sharing some insights with people that you are sitting next to. Or use SoMe to engage in a Twitter chat in an area of interest. We promise that others will be interested in what you have to say.

- Not very interested in others.

  Are you really not interested in others, or are you maybe worried about what others think of you? In your professional practice, it is essential that you are interested in people – take that interest in people into the discussions you have with people who are working in your field of practice. You may learn lots.

- Too busy, haven't got time.

  It is a busy life, but there is always time for short interactions whether they are in 'real' life or in social media. It doesn't take much to start building relationships, and you may find that the growth of your networks will save you time, as you will have people that you can go to for quick advice.

- How do I begin?

  Why not go back to activities 8.1 and 8.4 and choose one of the 'gaps' that you have identified. Then find a way to make a connection with that person or organisation.

- How do I choose what event to go to?

  What is of interest to you? What is important for your professional practice?

Finally, here are some tips to help you in successful networking.

- Know yourself and what you have to offer – skills, experiences, training, qualities, attributes – and be proud of them.
- Ask for support where you need it.
- Develop a network diagram and know where your gaps are and have a plan to fill them.
- Introduce yourself to others in a way that generates interest and is clear and concise and engaging.
- Speak to people outside of your comfort zone.
- Re-introduce yourself to people; don't wait for them to remember you.
- Be an active listener; remember people's names and what they do.
- Show that you care about people by the way you listen, and be polite and interested.
- Build your confidence so you can increase your own visibility.
- Nurture your network with follow-up calls.
- Return calls as soon as possible.
- Prepare for networking events to get the most out of them.
- If you ask for help from your network be straightforward and specific.

SUMMARY

Some key learning points from this chapter include:

- Networking is a lifelong process that enables you to extend your contacts, your knowledge-base, your support and your skills.
- There are multiple ways to network, all of which bring their own advantages and enable you to engage in ways that are most suitable for your personality type and your personal circumstances.
- Social media as a tool for networking bring immediate impact into your networks through engagement at a global level with practitioners, commentators, academics and others.

FURTHER RESOURCES

Barry, J. and Hardiker, N.R. (2012) 'Advancing nursing practice through social media: a global perspective'. *The Online Journal of Issues in Nursing*, 17(3): Manuscript 5.

A useful read that provides a coherent overview of the current context of social networking for nursing practice.

Taylor, R. (2013) 'Networking in primary health care: how connections can increase social capital'. *Primary Health Care*, 23(10): 34–40.

This continuing professional practice article succinctly addresses networking for professional practice within one setting – primary healthcare – but has wider implications for nursing practice.

 To access further resources related to this chapter, please visit the companion website at https://study.sagepub.com/taylor

REFERENCES

Albrecht, K. (2006) *Social Intelligence: The New Science of Success*. San Francisco: Jossey-Bass.

Baines, D. and Hale, C. (2004) 'Use network theory to develop services'. *Pharmaceutical Journal*, 272: 222–3.

Barry, J. and Hardiker, N.R. (2012) 'Advancing nursing practice through social media: a global perspective. *The Online Journal of Issues in Nursing*, 17(3): Manuscript 5.

Brady, A.M., Malone, A.M. and Fleming, S. (2009) 'A literature review of the individual and system factors that contribute to errors in nursing practice'. *Journal of Nursing Management*, 17(6): 679–97.

Buggy, C. (2006). 'Connecting up to the network'. *Professional Manager*, March: 26–8.

Carroll, T.L. (2005) 'Leadership skills and attributes of women and nurse executives: challenges for the 21st century'. *Nurse Administration Quarterly*, 29(2): 146.

Enterkin, J., Robb, E. and MacLaren, S. (2013) 'Clinical leadership for high quality care: developing future ward leaders'. *Journal of Nursing Management*, 21: 206–16.

Ferguson, C. (2013) 'Editorial: It's time for the nursing profession to leverage social media'. *Journal of Advanced Nursing*, 69(4): 745–7.

Field, J. (2008) *Social Capital*, 2nd edition. Oxford: Routledge.

Gladwell, M. (2002) *The Tipping Point*. New York: Abacus.

Griffey, H. (2009) *The Nurse Executives' Handbook: Leading the Business of Caring from Board to Ward*. London: Burdett Trust for Nursing/King's Fund.

Grossman, S.C. and Valiga, T.M. (2013) *The New Leadership Challenge: Creating the Future of Nursing*. Philadelphia: F A Davis Company.

Kaplan, A.M. and Haenlein, M. (2010) 'Users of the world, unite! The challenges and opportunities of social media'. *Business Horizons*, 53(1): 59–68.

Kalisch, B. and Aebersold, M. (2010) 'Interruptions in multitasking in nursing care'. *Journal of Quality Patient Safety*, 36(3): 126–32.

Koteyko, N., Hunt, D. and Gunter, B. (2015) 'Expectations in the field of the internet and health: an analysis of claims about social networking sites in clinical literature'. *Sociology of Health and Illness*, 37(3): 468–84.

Lawson, C. and Cowling, C. (2014) 'Social media: the next frontier for professional development in radiography'. *Radiography*, 21: 74–80.

Marshall, E.S. (2011) *Transformational Leadership in Nursing: From Expert Clinician to Influential Leader*. New York: Springer Publishing Company.

Nursing and Midwifery Council (2015) *The Code: Professional Standards of Practice and Behaviour for Nurses and Midwives*. London: NMC.

Piscotty, R., Voepel-Lewis, T., Lee, S., Annis, A., Lee, E. and Kalisch, B. (2015) 'Hold the phone: nurses, social media and patient care'. *Nursing*, 45(5): 64–7.

Putnam, R. (1995) 'Bowling alone: America's declining social capital'. *Journal of Democracy*, 6(1): 65–78.

Ressler, P.K. and Glazer, G. (2010) 'Legislative: nursing's engagement in health policy and healthcare through social media'. *The Online Journal of Issues in Nursing*, 16(1): 1–5.

Schmitt, T.L., Sims-Giddens, S.S. and Booth, R.G. (2012) 'Social media use in nursing education'. *Online Journal of Issues in Nursing*, 17(3): Manuscript 2.

Scott, C. and Hofmeyer, A. (2007) 'Networks and social capital: a relational approach to primary healthcare reform'. *Health Research Policy and Systems*, 5(9). DOI: 10.1186/1478-4505-5-9.

Taylor, R. (2013) 'Networking in primary health care: how connections can increase social capital'. *Primary Health Care*, 23(10): 34–40.

Watts, D.J. (2004) *Six Degrees: The Science of a Connected Age*. London: WW Norton and Company Ltd.

9 PREPARATION FOR TRANSITION TO LEADERSHIP IN QUALIFIED PRACTICE

Jayne Donaldson and Mike Sabin

Chapter learning outcomes

On completion of this chapter you will be able to:

- Recognise the need to develop your leadership skills from student nurse through the transition to being a registrant and beyond.
- Describe the types of leadership that could be effective in clinical practice.
- Demonstrate knowledge of the types of transitional support that you could access following registration as a nurse.

Key concepts

Clinical leadership and authenticity, collective leadership, authentic leadership, reality/transition shock, early careers

INTRODUCTION

Transition from being a student to a newly qualified nurse is possibly an area that you have thought about (depending on how far you are in your degree at the moment). You may feel a sense of excitement when you think about being out in practice as a qualified nurse. At the same time, you may also have some anxieties about this change in your role – don't worry, that is not unusual. In this chapter we offer an overview of some of the key issues associated with transition to professional practice, and discuss how you can prepare yourself for this period of change. We have included a list of resources which we hope will serve as a toolkit for your transition.

Nurses are increasingly being asked to develop and use leadership skills in their practice and yet it has been suggested that focused leadership development education is not always well embedded in the undergraduate nursing curriculum (Curtis et al., 2011). In this chapter, we stress the importance of leadership skills for nurses at every stage of their career, and that preparation for practice within pre-registration degrees and the transition into subsequent professional practice offers both a series of challenges and opportunities to reshape our understanding of, and commitment to, leadership in clinical practice.

Communication skills and leadership attributes which focus on openness and shared accountability contribute to improved outcomes for service users, particularly in terms of patient safety (Vogelsmeier et al., 2010; Williams and Reid, 2009). Reports into recent failures of healthcare organisations and suggested improvements in care, such as the Mid Staffordshire NHS Trust Inquiry (Francis, 2013), Improving the Safety of Patients in England (Berwick, 2013), the Vale of Leven Hospital Inquiry (MacLean, 2014) and the Keogh Mortality Review (Keogh, 2013) all identified leadership deficits within the organisational cultures and argued that the resulting values and normative behaviours in those situations created the conditions for what ensued (West et al., 2014). Middleton (2013) argues that leadership is an essential concept for undergraduate nurses to grasp so that they can begin to understand that their role as newly registered nurses will be one with a central focus on facilitating and leading positive change. Indeed, leadership skills, focused not only on clinical excellence, organisational efficiency and effectiveness but also on wider social justice, will be critical for challenging and addressing those societal inequalities that have adversely affected the health of those who receive your care. This requires that you develop leadership skills to become agents of change within healthcare to improve health outcomes in marginalised populations.

Viewed in this way, nursing leadership is not seen as an adjunct to care giving and care assurance, but rather as an integral part of these processes. However, Bagnall (2012) identifies that learning, teaching and assessment of leadership and team working concepts and practice are often squeezed out of undergraduate health curricula in preference for a greater focus on clinical patient care.

Activity 9.1

Consider your own experience of learning so far with regard to leadership.

- Where has your leadership learning been evidenced so far in your course?
- What impact has it had on the development of your leadership skills?

Given that nursing care is an essential component of healthcare provision and must be delivered by professionals with the optimum clinical skill, knowledge and professional values, then an understanding of nursing leadership becomes essential so as to ensure care is safe, effective and person-centred. In this context, learning how you could (and should) contribute to clinical, operational and professional leadership would appear to be one of the core principles of any professional education curriculum.

UNDERSTANDING THE PERCEPTIONS OF NEWLY REGISTERED NURSES AND THEIR PREPARATION FOR LEADERSHIP AND PATIENT CARE

How you perceive yourself in relation to 'leadership' will have a profound impact upon your professional practice. If leadership ability is considered to be something with which an individual is born, then your engagement with the concept within your education and development as a practitioner will be defined by whether you believe that you have this ability/potential or don't. Likewise, if that is true, your lecturers, mentors and supervisors should be focusing on facilitating and developing that leadership ability/potential in those students displaying such characteristics whilst simultaneously focusing on supporting 'followership' across the rest of the student body. Alternatively, if leadership potential exists in all of us, then the focus of the educational and development process changes fundamentally, along with individual and collective expectations as to who might (and should) adopt such roles. Further, accepting the idea that we all have a leadership role impacts directly upon how such skills and understanding will be embedded within professional practice.

When asked to think of leadership, you may cite concepts of power, hierarchy, self-belief, trustworthiness, goal orientation, influential behaviour and personality (Curtis et al., 2011). This perspective has been established, and perpetuated by classical literature, popular media and by some political and sociological theorists. The idea of a leadership 'birthright' continues to hold a surprisingly strong place in our culture, and any challenge to this orthodoxy requires a concerted approach linked to enhanced understanding of what leadership is, who provides and engages with it, and what role it should play in practice.

Kouzes and Posner (2006: 13) describe leadership as:

> an observable, learnable set of practices, not something mystical and ethereal that cannot be understood by ordinary people.

They argue that those with the desire to lead can significantly improve their abilities to do so if given the opportunity for feedback and practice. Therefore, leadership should not be seen as an inherent 'state' but as a set of practices that can be taught, nurtured and strengthened through education, practice and feedback. We also argue that 'leadership' and 'followership' are not independent or exclusive roles but are instead mutually dependant and supportive activities, each requiring knowledgeable and informed choice.

Not everyone will take this view and Gunter (2001: 105) has argued that:

> models of leadership are not neutral but are the product of enduring power structures in which there are attempts in different economic, historical, political and social contexts to determine what is and is not effective leadership.

As a student nurse it is important to continually consider and review what leadership means to you and your practice. In that context, the next key question is whether leadership is principally characterised by individual or collective action? Leadership should not necessarily be associated with holding a position of power (Thoms and Duffield, 2012), nor should it be associated with any particular title or pay scale. Leadership is not always a fixed or permanent 'position', but more a set of actions and consequences linked to an outcome or goal. Indeed, the concept of *collective leadership* proposes a model where leadership power is distributed to wherever expertise, capability and motivation sit within organisations (West et al., 2014). The aim of such an approach is to create an organisational context and professional culture in which all staff seek to take responsibility for high quality and compassionate care. West et al. (2014) argue that, in such a culture, roles of 'leadership' and 'followership' will shift depending on situational requirements as every member of staff has the potential to lead at different points in time, particularly when their expertise is relevant to the task in hand. Reciprocally, it is also important that all staff are equally focused on opportunities to enact good 'followership' behaviours, regardless of their position in the organisation or professional hierarchy.

Importantly, collective leadership should not be seen as some laissez-faire, diffusion of responsibility and accountability, but as a deliberately shared and enabling process that requires an active understanding of, and engagement with, the leadership practices and behaviours needed to develop and sustain excellent practice. As West et al. (2014: 8) state:

> Conscious, deliberate attention must be paid to enabling people at every level within the organisation to adopt leadership practices that nurture the cultures the NHS requires.

Leadership does not lie with or within the individual but in the relationship *between* individuals, and can be considered a process orientated towards social vision and change and not merely the achievement of organisational goals (Gunter, 2001). At the beginning of your professional nursing career, it is important that you see leadership both as a participative process within which all involved can play a role and as a mechanism through which new or previously unheard perspectives can influence the shaping and focus of our care. You can use this idea to legitimise your own contribution to clinical leadership whilst allowing space for you to hear and consider other perspectives. The new leader's ability to be effective in offering constructive challenge and being assertive in prioritising and leading high quality care outcomes comes not from their own individual personality style, but from a leadership context that facilitates such actions.

Despite the ideas presented above, it is important to understand that there is no single model of leadership in clinical service which has been *proven* to work best, so it is important that you gain an understanding of the various models of leadership and then consider how these are exhibited, and how they impact upon outcomes as you develop and progress through your career. Indeed, you may look to review, use and evaluate more than one model of leadership depending upon your stage of career and the type of post and role you hold.

BARRIERS TO DEVELOPING LEADERSHIP POTENTIAL

Whilst nursing as a profession remains strongly gendered, with only around 10% of the profession being male (NMC, 2014), this has not necessarily conferred advantage regarding leadership influence for women, with a disproportionate number of those men occupying senior roles. Bolden et al. (2011) identify that leadership has been defined stereotypically as 'masculine' and associated with control and command. Schedlitzki and Edwards (2014) suggest that despite more recent shifts in both the number of women in leadership positions and gender-influenced conceptions of leadership, the predominant leadership culture is still highly gendered. It is important to recognise that barriers to participating in leadership roles are not limited to gender, but involve ethnicity, age, social class, education and sexual orientation. The interplay between these factors is complex and shifting, particularly if considered from different cultural perspectives.

Certainly, traditional conceptions of the nursing role have tended to emphasise the 'supportive', feminised role of the nurse within a medically dominated, masculine infrastructure. However, there are also strong historical female role models (Nightingale, Seacole) and many current male and female leaders (e.g. Gail Adams, Head of Nursing, Unison; Yinglen Butt, Deputy Chief Nurse, Guy's and St. Thomas' Foundation Trust; Maurice Devine, Assistant Director, Ireland's Department of Health and Social Care Clinical Education Centre) who offer an alternative perspective and one that may be a stimulus for awakening and realising leadership potential amongst those who might not otherwise have had such exposure. It is these perspectives that are so important to you as a student nurse who will be making the transition to qualified practice – you will need to reflect on them and make your own decisions about how best to take forward your own leadership practice.

Activity 9.2

Write a short piece on your personal view of yourself as a leader, and your readiness (or otherwise) for leadership in clinical practice.

If you are coming towards the end of your degree and getting ready for that transition to qualified practice, an honest reflection which acknowledges your strengths is a good starting point for developing a view on your own leadership development needs.

TRANSITION TO PROFESSIONAL PRACTICE: MAXIMISING LEADERSHIP POTENTIAL IN EARLY CAREERS

It is at the point of transition into professional practice as a registered nurse that you may experience a significant step change in your perception of competence and confidence in this area (Ekstrom and Idvall, 2015). The concept of 'Transition Shock' (Duchscher, 2009) built upon the 'Reality Shock' theory developed by Kramer (1974) describes how new graduates practising for the first time in their full professional role are confronted by a range of physical, intellectual, emotional, developmental and socio-cultural challenges as they transition from their 'student' role and identity to that of the registered practitioner.

Much has been made of the role of students as 'change agents', bringing new perspectives and challenging orthodoxies in both education and clinical practice (Ion et al., 2015). Whilst there is little doubt that both new staff and students bring an external perspective to established practice, Pullen (2003) identified that, for the most part, the focus of the student lies in 'fitting in' to an established team, rather than challenging the norms of practice. Is this something that you have felt when you have been in clinical practice? There is a risk that this need to assimilate becomes the key driver for student and newly registered nurse behaviour, rather than fostering early leadership skills, particularly when faced with challenging situations (Ion et al., 2015).

Activity 9.3

Reflect on how you felt when you started your most recent clinical placement.

- Did you aim to 'fit in'?
- Did you feel able to constructively challenge practice or ask questions?
- What were the key issues for you in demonstrating leadership within this context?

As you were reflecting, you may have identified some of the issues that Lekan et al. (2011) found in their study. They trialled a transitional leadership support model, and explored students' perceptions of their leadership capabilities. They identified low leadership self-efficacy, challenges in managing the 'credibility gap' when engaging with other staff, and concerns regarding accountability in delegation and supervision as key issues for new staff. Watts and Gordon (2012) note that there may well be a gap between educational preparation in nursing and the reality of practice in complex clinical settings, leaving nurses unprepared for effective frontline leadership. There is considerable debate (not confined to nursing) as to whether any form of educational programme can adequately prepare students for every situation that may arise during the transition into professional practice (Valiga and Champagne, 2010). Duchscher (2009) identified that many new graduates entering the workplace struggled to maintain their own visions for practice that they had built up and consolidated during their pre-registration education and which they believed were a basic requirement of their professional role. This feeling of being unable to effectively challenge less than optimal practice was demoralising and, in turn, challenged their own sense of themselves as emerging professional leaders. These statements are not intended to concern you. Rather, they are made to raise awareness so that you can think about how you apply your learning in clinical practice, how you further develop your leadership skills, and so that you acknowledge that the development of these skills does not take place quickly but is the result of ongoing development.

In that context, and recognising that students and newly registered practitioners may find the integration of leadership practice within their role challenging, it is vital that there is a 'scaffolding' structure in place to support, nurture and critique that practice as it develops during the pre-registration preparation and, perhaps most importantly, during transition into early professional practice. The presence or absence of such support and the provision of protected reflective learning 'space' within which to practice leadership skills impacts in turn on successful transition (Carlin and Duffy, 2013; Magnusson et al., 2014). The key areas of support argued to enhance the experience of transition into professional practice involve a strategic, operational and individual professional focus on leadership through four interconnected components which we'll look at in turn (see Figure 9.1).

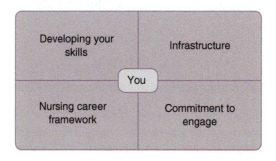

Figure 9.1   Support for transition into professional practice

PRE-REGISTRATION PREPARATION IN DEVELOPING YOUR LEADERSHIP SKILLS

Pullen (2003), Lekan et al. (2011), Middleton (2013) and Brown et al. (2015) have all emphasised the importance of a scheme of leadership education integrated throughout the pre-registration curriculum which emphasises and models the relationship with clinical/professional practice. The Nursing and Midwifery Council's *Standards for Pre-registration Nursing Education* (NMC, 2010) set out the expectations for all pre-registration nursing programmes within the UK, with competencies organised in the four domains with a particular focus on leadership, management and team working (see the introduction to this book). Leadership is identified by the regulator as one of the core professional domains and, whilst field-specific examples of leadership competencies are identified, the generic standard for competence in this domain is:

> All nurses must be professionally accountable and use clinical governance processes to maintain and improve nursing practice and standards of healthcare. They must be able to respond autonomously and confidently to planned and uncertain situations, managing themselves and others effectively. They must create and maximise opportunities to improve services. They must also demonstrate the potential to develop further management and leadership skills during their period of preceptorship and beyond. (NMC, 2010: 29)

This statement makes clear the importance of the relationship between leadership and professional practice, emphasising that the focus and purpose of educational development for clinical leadership are to enable and ensure the highest standards of care to clients and to maximise support to the healthcare team in the delivery of that care.

It is important to recognise that within each of the four competency domains there are elements of leadership that you need to demonstrate and develop throughout your pre-registration degree. The Nursing and Midwifery Council (NMC) also emphasises that achievement of these is not the end point, but the *springboard* into that period of transition to a qualified nurse and beyond. Within your own pre-registration degree, you will have been developing your leadership skills through your learning and understanding of leadership within the theory and practice elements of your programme, and it is essential that you see these opportunities as integral to your developing professional competence rather than as an *add-on* to your clinical competence. Recognising your own values, strengths and areas for leadership development will help you identify how you currently practise, and encourage you to reflect forward into your qualified practitioner role. Greater self-awareness in these situations may create anxiety but, equally, it will be important in providing the platform upon which appropriate leadership behaviours can be developed and supported. In this way, the experience of 'transition shock' explored earlier can be significantly mitigated by focusing on developing your practice and confidence in these areas, and preparing for that shift in focus before you encounter this in reality.

A SUPERVISORY/MENTORING INFRASTRUCTURE WHICH IS FOCUSED ON BUILDING AND VALUING THIS PILLAR OF PRACTICE

A key factor in driving and supporting leadership awareness, understanding and engagement will be the quality of the mentorship, preceptorship and supervision which you as a student or newly registered nurse experience. As you transition from student to registrant, there will be a growing understanding of 'Who am I?', i.e. an understanding of yourself and 'Who I want to become'; and also a greater appreciation of 'Who are we?', i.e. of collective values within the clinical team, the organisation in which you work and the profession as a whole (Fachin and Davel, 2015; Kreiner et al., 2006). Opportunities to practise, observe and model leadership skills lead to a greater self-efficacy in nurses' leadership behaviours (Watts and Gordon, 2012; Hendricks et al., 2010).

Research shows that student nurses value relationship qualities such as effective communication and approachability highly in the people supporting them to bridge the gap between student and qualified practice (Curtis et al., 2011). Phillips et al. (2013), when exploring the relationship between pre-registration employment and subsequent transition into registered employment, found that post-registration institutional work factors appeared to be stronger predictors of successful transition than pre-registration employment factors. Assistance in dealing with complex patients, orientation to a new environment and respect from colleagues were the best predictors for successful transition.

The presence of positive role models will be important in helping emerging leaders to model their own leadership practice, but Bjorklund and Holt (2012) suggested that such examples may not always be readily available to staff transitioning into their new role. Recognising the need to strengthen preceptorship arrangements and to provide practical support to both preceptors and newly registered practitioners, the Flying Start NHS® programme (Stewart and Barber, 2011; Upton et al., 2012) was established in 2006 in Scotland as the national online development programme for all newly qualified nurses, midwives and allied health professionals. It seeks to provide support for both new registrants and their mentors in developing skills and building confidence during the first year of registered practice. This infrastructure provides a developmental framework within which the newly registered nurse can explore their developing role and draw upon available resources to support their ongoing career. Similar initiatives have now been taken forward in the other countries of the UK. In Northern Ireland, the Northern Ireland Practice and Education Council for Nursing and Midwifery (NIPEC) launched its Preceptorship Framework (NIPEC/DSSPS, 2013). The mini-website provides guidance for new registrants, their preceptors and managers to support transition, and promotes a structured period of transition for new registrants, during which they work with a preceptor who acts as a role model, helping to enhance their confidence, competence and critical decision-making. In 2014, the Welsh Government/NHS Wales published its *Core Principles for Preceptorship* document and, in England, the Department of Health (DH, 2010) published their *Preceptorship Framework for Newly Registered Nurses, Midwives and Allied Health Professionals*. These were aimed more at those managing preceptorship programmes at Trust or Board level, and outlined the elements of good preceptorship practice and suggested outcome measures to realise benefits.

A NURSING CAREER AND DEVELOPMENTAL FRAMEWORK WITH LEADERSHIP AS A CORE PILLAR

If we accept that leadership skills are central to professional practice, then these require to be embedded not just within educational preparation and local induction and support arrangements, but also in wider strategic workforce development, planning and commissioning. Both the UK government and the health and care departments of the devolved governments have identified leadership as a particular area of focus since *Modernising Nursing Careers* (DH, 2006). The emergence of the National Leadership Unit in Scotland and the NHS Leadership Academy in England is testimony to a strategic focus in these areas, as calls to strengthen the focus on clinical leadership continue to be made amid perceptions of weakness in these fields. Alongside this strategic commitment, a number of supportive developmental tools have been launched to provide guidance to new practitioners and those supporting early leadership development.

Within Scotland, the *Post Registration Career Development Framework* (NHS Education for Scotland, 2014) provides guidance to practitioners and managers.

Information box 9.1: The four pillars of professional practice (NHS Education for Scotland, 2014)

- Clinical practice.
- Facilitation of learning.
- Leadership.
- Evidence, research and development.

The NHS Education for Scotland (2014) framework identifies key aspects of practice which are transferable across disciplines and seeks to support a greater consistency of approach across different professional and speciality groups. As with the other pillars, the leadership pillar demonstrates how clinical and professional leadership can be articulated at each of the different levels of the career framework, supporting practitioners to understand where they might be on the development continuum and to guide their professional development. As you transition from student to newly registered practitioner and onwards in your career, it is important that you are able to benchmark your own practice against the expectations of the role you will be taking on. This is just as true for leadership as it is for facilitating learning or for clinical practice skills.

A COMMITMENT BY THE INDIVIDUAL LEARNER/ PRACTITIONER TO ENGAGE WITH LEADERSHIP AS A CORE ELEMENT OF THEIR PRACTICE

The NMC holds the statutory responsibility for the regulation of all nurses and midwives in the UK and requires all registered practitioners to demonstrate professional behaviours that are described in the various standards and codes set down by the regulator. Whilst the principal focus of regulation is upon professional practice, we all undertake that practice within wider organisations and healthcare systems. Indeed, the NMC Code states that:

You should be a model of integrity and leadership for others to aspire to. (NMC, 2015a: 15)

Provide leadership to make sure people's wellbeing is protected and to improve their experiences of the healthcare system. (NMC, 2015a: 18)

It is important to understand that, as a registered nurse, you will have an intrinsic responsibility to improve patient experience and outcomes by: contributing to the leadership process at an individual level; developing and facilitating the leadership capacity and capability of colleagues; and acting as a change agent in leading and influencing wider organisational systems. Nurses need to have the leadership skills to know when and how to raise concerns, such as through whistleblowing policies and procedures, as well as to challenge care practices through developing research findings, using evidence-based practice and quality improvement methodologies. Therefore, it is essential that you develop these leadership skills now and also continually refresh and strengthen these as core requirements for your future professional roles and career.

Activity 9.4

Imagine that you are going for your first job interview as a newly qualified nurse. Think about the leadership qualities that you have developed in your time on your course.

- How will you articulate these to the interview panel – both within your application and at interview?
- What would you like to strengthen and develop, especially in your first year as a newly qualified nurse?

Your ongoing development as a leader will be essential in order that you can respond to a healthcare environment which will undergo ongoing change in its structure, organisation and individual career/professional requirements. Employees are increasingly aware that career success is dependent upon self-awareness and also the capacity and willingness to be flexible and responsive to change. As Clarke (2009: 23) states:

Mind-sets and behaviours, such as lifelong learning, flexibility, adaptability, self-awareness, networking and career planning, help build career assets and thus support ongoing employability and long-term career success.

One driver for a refreshed focus on leadership within our professional roles is the introduction of revalidation by the NMC. Revalidation seeks to provide a focus on our values, competence and professionalism and how those are reflected in, and respond to, those with whom we work and amongst the wider workforce. The NMC (2015b) has stated that revalidation will promote good practice by introducing new requirements for registrants to focus on:

- up-to-date practice and professional development;
- reflection on the professional standards of practice and behaviour as set out in the Code; and
- engagement in professional discussions with other registered nurses or midwives.

As students and as NMC registrants, reflective practice will have been a core aspect of your professional development and, in the context of revalidation, there is an opportunity for you to not only engage in active reflection about your professional role and contribution to care delivery, but also to open up your individual professional practice, values and competence to other colleagues. Indeed, the NMC Code sets an explicit requirement to 'Share your skills, knowledge and experience for the benefit of people receiving care and your colleagues' (NMC, 2015a: 8). These activities are not only central to the revalidation process and its focus on assuring individual professional practice, but also clearly support a collective commitment to a distributed model of professional clinical leadership practice.

SUMMARY

Some key learning points in this chapter include:

- Leadership is a core 'pillar' of professional practice and deserves (and requires) the same focus in your learning and development as clinical, educational and research skills.
- Leadership is a collective as well as an individual endeavour.
- Effective leadership comes from a combination of strategic, developmental and professional commitment.

FURTHER RESOURCES

The Healthcare Leadership Model and the Clinical Leadership Competency Model – in the NHS Leadership Academy (2013) (available at: www.leadershipacademy.nhs.uk/)

The Edward Jenner Programme – in the NHS Leadership Academy (2013) (available at: www.leadershipacademy.nhs.uk/)

For staff beginning to work towards more formal clinical leadership and management roles such as Charge Nurse or Team Leader, further structured development work such as the NIPEC Leading Teams website (www.nipec.hscni.net/welcome-to-the-nipec-leading-teams-website/) and the NES Leading Better Care resources (available at: www.leadingbettercare.scot.nhs.uk/) provide learning materials and self-assessment tools to support development.

To access further resources related to this chapter, please visit the companion website at https://study.sagepub.com/taylor

REFERENCES

Bagnall, P. (2012) *Facilitators and Barriers to Leadership and Quality Improvement*. The King's Fund Junior Doctor Project. London: King's Fund, pp. 1–32.

Berwick D (2013) A promise to learn – a commitment to act Improving the Safety of Patients in England. Department of Health (England). Available at: www.gov.uk/government/publications/berwick-review-into-patient-safety. Accessed 16/06/2016).

Bjorklund, R.L. and Holt, S. (2012) 'Overcoming barriers to participation in diverse strategic decision-making groups: a leadership perspective'. *International Journal of Business and Management*, 7(6): 49–58.

Bolden, R., Hawkins, B., Gosling, J. and Taylor, S. (2011) *Exploring Leadership: Individual, Organisational and Societal Perspectives*. Oxford: Oxford University Press.

Brown, A., Crookes, P. and Dewing, J. (2015) 'Clinical leadership development in a pre-registration nursing curriculum: what the profession has to say about it'. *Nurse Education Today*, 36: 105–11.

Carlin, A. and Duffy, K. (2013) 'Newly qualified staff's perceptions of senior charge nurse roles'. *Nursing Management*, 20(7): 24–30.

Clarke, M. (2009) 'Plodders, pragmatists, visionaries and opportunists: career patterns and employability'. *Development and Learning in Organizations*, 14(1): 8–28.

Curtis, E.A., Sheerin, F.K. and de Vries, J. (2011) 'Developing leadership in nursing: the impact of education and training'. *British Journal of Nursing*, 20(6): 344–52.

Department of Health (2006) *Modernising Nursing Careers*. London: DH.

Department of Health (2010) *Preceptorship Framework for Newly Registered Nurses, Midwives and Allied Health Professionals*. London: DH. Available at: www.cmft.nhs.uk/published/UserUpload/file/DoH%20Preceptorship%20%20AHPs,%20Nurses%20Midwifery.pdf. Accessed 16/06/2016.

Duchscher, J.E.B. (2009) 'Transition shock: the initial stage of role adaptation for newly graduated registered nurses'. *Journal of Advanced Nursing*, 65(5): 1103–13.

Ekstrom, L. and Idvall, E. (2015) 'Being a team leader: newly registered nurses relate their experiences'. *Journal of Nursing Management*, 23: 75–86.

Fachin, F.F. and Davel, E. (2015) 'Reconciling contradictory paths: identity play and work in career transition'. *Journal of Organizational Change Management*, 28(3): 369–92.

Francis, R. (2013) *Report of the Mid Staffordshire NHS Foundation Trust Public Inquiry: Executive Summary* (Vol. 947). London: The Stationery Office.

Gunter, H. (2001) 'Critical approaches to leadership in education'. *Journal of Educational Enquiry*, 2(2): 94–108.

Hendricks, J.M., Cope, V.C. and Harris, M. (2010) 'A leadership program in an undergraduate nursing course in Western Australia: building leaders in our midst', *Nurse Education Today*, 30: 252–57.

Ion, R., Smith, K., Nimmo, S., Rice, A.M. and McMillan, L. (2015) 'Factors influencing student nurse decisions to report poor practice witnessed while on placement'. *Nurse Education Today*, 35(7): 900–5.

Keogh, Sir Bruce (2013) *Review into the Quality of Care and Treatment Provided by 14 Hospital Trusts in England: Overview Report*. London: DH.

Kouzes, J and Posner, B. (2006) *The Student Leadership Practices Inventory*. San Francisco: Jossey-Bass.

Kramer, M. (1974) *Reality Shock: Why Nurses Leave Nursing*. St Louis: C.V. Mosby.

Kreiner, G.E., Hollensbe, E.C. and Sheep, M.L. (2006) 'Where is the "me" in the "we"? Identity work and the search for optimal balance'. *Academy of Management Journal*, 49(5): 1031–57.

Lekan, D.A., Corazzini, K.N., Gilliss, C.L. and Bailey, D.E. (2011) 'Clinical leadership development in accelerated baccalaureate nursing students: an education innovation'. *Journal of Professional Nursing*, 27(4): 202–14.

MacLean, The Rt Hon. Lord (Chair) (2014) *The Vale of Leven Hospital Inquiry Report.* Edinburgh: Scottish Government. [Online] Available at www.valeoflevenhospitalinquiry.org/Report/j156505.pdf. Accessed 18/08/15.

Magnusson, C., Westwood, S., Ball, E., Curtis, K., Evans, K., Horton, K., Johnson, M. and Allan, H. (2014) *An Investigation into Newly Qualified Nurses' Ability to Recontextualise Knowledge to Allow Them to Delegate and Supervise Care (AaRK).* University of Surrey/GNC for England and Wales Trust.

Middleton, R. (2013) 'Active learning and leadership in an undergraduate curriculum: how effective is it for student learning and transition to practice?'. *Nurse Education in Practice*, 13: 83–8.

NHS Education for Scotland (2014) *Post-Registration Career Development Framework for Nurses, Midwives and Allied Health Professions.* Edinburgh: NHS Education for Scotland. [Online] Available at www.careerframework.nes.scot.nhs.uk. Accessed 12/9/2016.

Nursing and Midwifery Council (2010) *Standards for Pre-registration Nursing Education.* London: NMC. Available at: www.nmc.org.uk/standards/additional-standards/standards-for-pre-registration-nursing-education/. Accessed 16/06/2016.

Nursing and Midwifery Council (2014) *Equality and Diversity Annual Report 2014.* London: NMC. [Online] Available at www.nmc.org.uk/globalassets/sitedocuments/annual_reports_and_accounts/the-equality-and-diversity-annual-report---english-january-2015.pdf.

Nursing and Midwifery Council (2015a) *The Code: Professional Standards of Practice and Behaviour for Nurses and Midwives.* London: NMC. [Online] Available at www.nmc.org.uk/globalassets/sitedocuments/nmc-publications/revised-new-nmc-code.pdf. Accessed 12/9/2016.

Nursing and Midwifery Council (2015b) *Revalidation.* London: NMC. [Online] Available at www.nmc.org.uk/standards/revalidation. Accessed 12/9/2016.

Northern Ireland Practice and Education Council for Nursing and Midwifery (NIPEC)/Department of Health Social Services and Public Safety (DHSSPS) (2013) *Preceptorship Framework for Nursing, Midwifery and Specialist Community Public Health Nursing in Northern Ireland.* NIPEC/DHSSPS. Available at: www.nipec.hscni.net/guiding-principles-for-preceptorship-docs-2/. Accessed 16/06/2016.

Phillips, C., Esterman, A., Smith, C. and Kenny, A. (2013) 'Predictors of successful transition to registered nurse'. *Journal of Advanced Nursing*, 69(6): 1314–22.

Pullen ML (2003) 'Developing clinical leadership skills in student nurses', *Nurse Education Today*, 23(1):34–9.

Schedlitzki, D. and Edwards, G. (2014) *Studying Leadership: Traditional and Critical Approaches.* London: SAGE.

Stewart, J. and Barber, L. (2011) 'A Flying Start for the Newly Qualified'. *Nursing Times*, 107(19/20): 19.

Thoms, D. and Duffield, C. (2012) 'Clinical leadership'. In: Chang, E. and Daly, J. (eds) *Transitions in Nursing.* Sydney: Elsevier, pp. 225–34.

Upton, D., Upton, P. and Erol, R. (2012) *Evaluation of the Key Characteristics which Support the Completion of Flying Start NHS® in NHS Scotland – Final Report for NHS Education for*

Scotland. [Online] Available at www.flyingstart.scot.nhs.uk/media/71080/university%20 of%20worcester%20flying%20start%20nhs%20report%202012.pdf. Accessed 12/9/2016.

Valiga, T.M. and Champagne, M. (2010) 'Creating the future of nursing education: challenges and opportunities'. In: Cowen, P.S. and Moorhead, S. (eds) *Current Issues in Nursing*, 8th edition. St Louis: Mosby Elsevier, pp. 75–83.

Vogelsmeier, A., Scott-Cawiezell, J., Miller, B. and Griffith, S. (2010) 'Influencing leadership perceptions of patient safety through just culture training'. *Journal of Nursing Care Quality*, 25: 288–94.

Watts, C. and Gordon, J. (2012) *Leadership and Pre-registration Nurse Education – Literature Review Included as Part of the Willis Commission 'Technical Papers'*. Available at: www.willis commission.org.uk/__data/assets/pdf_file/0009/480087/Leadership_and_pre-registration_ nurse_education.pdf. Accessed 16/06/2016.

West, M., Eckert, R., Steward, K. and Pasmore, B. (2014) *Developing Collective Leadership for Health Care*. London: The King's Fund.

Williams, M. and Reid, J. (2009) 'Patient safety: leading improvement'. *Nursing Management*, 16: 30–4

10 HARNESSING YOUR SKILLS AS A FUTURE LEADER

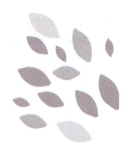

Role models in action

Brian Webster-Henderson

With thanks to Dave Ferguson, Debbie Carrick-Sen, Michael J. Brown, Juliet McArthur, Colette Ferguson and Tracy Humphrey

---

Chapter learning outcomes

In this chapter you will be able to:

- Explore the concept of *professional* leadership.
- Have the opportunity to learn from the narratives of some nursing leaders in the UK.
- Listen to the collective voice of those nursing leaders and identify common thoughts on leadership skills that you can aspire to.
- Consider how you can learn from 'role models' and adapt your own leadership potential.

Key concepts

Professional leadership, role models, collective voice, leadership narrative, advice

---

INTRODUCTION

This chapter introduces you to a number of leaders within the nursing profession. Six telephone or face-to-face interviews were conducted with leaders to gain an understanding of their career trajectories, the leadership influences on them as professionals, and to hear their advice for you as developing leaders. All the leaders interviewed gave their consent to share their personal stories and had the opportunity to read through the transcript of the interview before sharing it with you in this chapter. Finally, the chapter draws out some key messages in an analysis of their collective thoughts.

LEADERSHIP INTERVIEWS

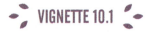

VIGNETTE 10.1

Dave Ferguson MBE, Consultant Nurse Cornerstone Health, England

Career trajectory

'I am a consultant nurse at Cornerstone Health in England. I have had a career in nursing that spans 36 years working in both community learning disability settings and in academia. I commenced my nursing career within an inpatient learning disability setting and then moved into the community. That's where the bulk of my career has been – working as a charge nurse and then as a clinical nurse specialist with learning disability clients who also had mental health issues.

I then took up a post at the University of Southampton as an academic and worked there for 12 years as an academic/practitioner, with the practice part of my role as a consultant nurse. I moved from there to the University of Hertfordshire and then progressed to my current role which is working with clients with cognitive impairments.'

What do you see as the influences that have inspired your professional leadership?

'I immediately think of role models. Three people come to mind – role models that I have worked with and I looked up to. One was a charge nurse, one was a director of operations and one was a senior lecturer. On reflection, they engaged with their staff, they knew their staff and worked with them. As role models they all had a vision and took staff with them in their ideas and thinking around quality patient care. They had an ability to empower me. I believe they saw my potential as a professional and used their skills to motivate, encourage and progress this to advantage. I also recall that these individuals all believed passionately in what they did.

I believe role models are still around and it's important that as professionals we can identify them and learn from them. One of my previous student nurses is now a senior member of staff where I work and it's inspiring to see her strengths and how she works with staff.

As a nurse, I do try to be like the role models I learned from. Nursing to me is more than a career; I still believe it is a vocation. That may not be a popular or contemporary thought but as a professional ... that's how I view it. I never came into nursing thinking I would get to this stage in my career, but I came to nursing because I passionately believed I could offer something to clients with a learning disability.

In 2013 I was awarded an MBE in the Queen's Honours list for my services to nursing and healthcare. I was shocked ... a complete surprise and felt why me? I am just doing my job ... But I feel immensely proud and honoured ... when it eventually sunk in ... I felt privileged and proud.

As well as role models that I recall in the past, I would also say that some of the people I work with currently also inspire me – the clients, the families and the carers. To live the lives they do live and how they overcome great barriers either in health or in services always inspires me in my professional identity and endorses me to do the job I do.

I enjoy working with nurses who want to provide the best care they can – they do exist in nursing, irrespective of what the press say and that inspires me. Their vision is about the best-evidenced based care they can give – that's my drive also.'

What advice would you provide to student nurses in supporting them to develop their leadership styles and skills?

'People need to get a range of clinical experiences, working with different patient groups. I would also suggest that where appropriate, project work, project management is really important too.

Getting a leadership mentor or coach is important and can be really useful to individual development.

Try to shadow "leaders" – people that inspire you: a staff nurse, a charge nurse – people that you look up to. You can learn a lot by watching others!

Having some idea of where you want your future career to go is an important part of the journey.

Learning your craft ... the craft of nursing is important also.

I think it's also important early on in your career to have a vision for the profession of nursing, the profession you have chosen to work in. This inspires creative thinking, a focus to be excellent and provide leadership.

Finally, I would encourage any student, to be inspired by other students – your peers – we can learn so much from each other, irrespective of the stage we are at in our career.'

· ·

VIGNETTE 10.2

Professor Debbie Carrick-Sen, Florence Nightingale Foundation Clinical Professor in Nursing and Midwifery Research: University of Birmingham and Heart of England NHS Foundation Trust

Career trajectory

'I think it's fair to say I have had a pretty unconventional career pathway. I am a nurse and a midwife and have used knowledge and skills related to both during my whole career – this has been really important to me.

After qualifying as a midwife, I worked in a clinical academic role for two years with 50% of my time as a clinical midwife and 50% of my time in clinical research. In its time (1990) this really was quite unique in our profession and quite ground breaking.

I've held a number of other joint clinical academic roles where I combined my passions for clinical practice and clinical research, including managing a research midwifery team and leading a clinical research environment within a clinical research facility, and then had responsibility for clinical teaching in the clinical setting with a focus on applied research.

I also designed, developed and led a master's programme in clinical research and leadership at the University of Newcastle. This was a unique programme that really emphasised the importance of professional leadership in research.

As my clinical roles developed, I became Head of Nursing and Midwifery Research in a very large acute hospital trust in Newcastle upon Tyne. Throughout my career, I have always supported and engaged in my own research – this started two years post qualifying as a midwife. I think on reflection this was probably a rarity but was progressed by my own sense of determination.

Throughout my career I have always believed that it is important to publish in journals and for our professional voice to be heard by others – so I have published, supervised doctoral and master's students and achieved success in obtaining research grants – irrespective of the role I had.'

What do you see as the influences that have inspired your professional leadership?

'I have four key points to share on this:

1. Support and encouragement from other colleagues has been really important – this was mainly from medical staff due to the research roles I had but their understanding, skills and passion for the research I was involved in were inspirational.
2. My success onto the Royal College of Nursing Political Leadership programme inspired me to learn a lot. I learned about politics with a big "P" and a small "p" as well as learning a lot about myself as a professional and as an individual. In relation to self, I discovered that it doesn't matter how much you know or how much passion and insight you have – you can't drive something on your own – you have to engage with others and get others on board. I have also had the privilege of undertaking the Florence Nightingale Executive Scholarship programme, which was a pivotal and life-changing part of my career. It also helped consolidate my learning about myself and interactions with others. The more your career progresses, the more you realise that skills such as negotiating, persuading, being passionate and articulate – are all really important in everything you do. The higher you get, the fewer people there are to draw on – so leadership skills are really important the more your career develops: awareness of knowing others and realising that I have to adapt to others' styles of leadership and not expect everyone to adapt to mine!
3. Access mentorship – I have accessed mentorship over the last 10–12 years. Not always in nursing, not always in my own organisation – but the people I have received mentorship from have provided me with sound advice and challenged me to reach higher. I approached them for mentorship, so I would encourage other nurses and midwives to look for mentorship early on and use those mentors as a sounding board – to challenge practice and approaches to care. Coaching is equally important to help manage difficult environments and questions.
4. Personal characteristics – determination, persistence and belief in self and the issues of the profession! Nurses and midwives make a valuable contribution to research but I have always believed that this is best in the clinical setting. Being

a clinical professor is a challenging role, the research and evidence generated is practice focused and it requires momentum and resilience. Self-awareness is a key part of leadership – it helps you identify your strengths and weaknesses and allows you to develop.'

What advice would you provide to student nurses in supporting them to develop their leadership styles and skills?

'Learn to understand yourself before you begin to influence and negotiate with others.

Request mentorship – it won't come to you, you have to find it. Think outside the box!

Look for and apply for all opportunities you see – including formal leadership pro-grammes. Find out – investigate – there's loads out there.

Don't get hung up if it's not been done before because *leaders lay the new ground for others to tread*! Sometimes laying new ground and direction in our profession is pivotal to success.'

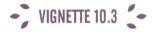

VIGNETTE 10.3

Professor Michael J. Brown, Professor/Nurse Consultant in Learning Disabilities, Edinburgh Napier University

Career trajectory

'I qualified in 1984 as a registered nurse for mental defectives (RNMD), which we now refer to as learning disabilities. I worked as a staff nurse within an inpatient paediatric learning disabilities unit before moving on to work within a male locked ward.

I then progressed into general nursing, qualifying in 1986 and undertook a number of staff nurse roles, mainly focused in male medical admissions and high dependency.

I then returned to learning disability nursing and progressed my career within commu-nity health settings whilst also going to university to achieve my degree in health sciences. Within community health services I held roles as a community nurse, practice teacher, service manager and in practice development, and progressed my learning with an MSc in politics and policy.

Following this I worked as a clinical nurse specialist, then in the Chief Nursing Officer's Department within government and on to a project lead role within the Public Health Insti-tute for Scotland.

I then went on to complete a PhD and worked in joint roles in practice and the university; senior lecturer/nurse consultant, reader/nurse consultant and finally clinical professor/nurse consultant.

On reflection I have had a really varied and rewarding career in a range of environments whilst also further developing my academic and research knowledge and skills.'

What do you see as the influences that have inspired your professional leadership?

'Firstly people – role models who have been hugely influential and powerful. They were generous with their time and ideas and have helped create the vision of what is possible.

They encouraged me to go and do it – even though I may not have always have believed in myself or had a fully formed vision of what I was going to do. I was encouraged around my innovation, new ideas, scanning the horizon and ability to encourage and motivate others. I think I now recognise the potential in others because that's what these nurse leaders did for me. So role models are key – I would suggest that you cannot underestimate the influence they have and the support they can offer.

In addition I think the lack of value placed on people working with learning disabilities has motivated me to want to provide the best possible care and quality of care I can. As a researcher I am driven to provide an evidence base to increase the quality of care, impact and value that we as professionals can provide to this population.'

What advice would you provide to student nurses in supporting them to develop their leadership styles and skills?

'Be clear about your own values and what motivates you to provide good patient care. Don't compromise on those values ... If you want to be popular – go find a job in a pub!

Find role models – people that you look up to and learn from them. Make an effort to ask to see them, sit with them and learn from their experience. You need to be slightly bold – make contact with them – prepare yourself before you go and speak to them, do a bit of background thinking so you can make best use of their time. Listen – and then reflect – then plan.

No one else has a responsibility for your career – you do, so personal ownership is pivotal and you need to be in this for the long haul; it won't happen overnight.

When you see opportunities – just go for them.

Don't get despondent if your ideas don't lead to the outcome you wanted – nothing is ever wasted – it will be of use at some point.'

. . . .

VIGNETTE 10.4

Dr Juliet McArthur, Chief Nurse in Research and Development, NHS Lothian/Lecturer in Clinical Academic Research, University of Edinburgh

Career trajectory

'I have been qualified since 1986 having decided at age 11 to become a nurse.

When I qualified I had undertaken my student management placement in a medical and haematology ward and so worked there for around nine months. I would say that this was one of the best clinical environments I ever worked in within my career – mainly due to the role model of the ward sister.

From there I moved to an acute surgical environment as a staff nurse and then was promoted to a senior staff nurse within a relatively quick period.

I felt my clinical knowledge base was not as strong as I wanted it to be, so I went to undertake some continuing professional development in critical care full time for six months. I stayed on in surgery then undertook a master's degree in nursing and health studies (1991–1993) part time. During this the concept of clinical audit was introduced within the NHS. A post came up in audit which I then was successful in achieving.

The research skills that I had been developing as a postgraduate student inspired me to want to progress further.

I was asked by the then Director of Nursing to work in practice development and lead this within the hospital. This prompted me to undertake a postgraduate certificate in education (2001–2003) and subsequently led to my progression focusing on research. I have held several roles as a lead practitioner in research until my current role as Chief Nurse in Research and Development where I have been since 2012. During this time I was also offered an honorary fellowship at the University of Edinburgh and completed my PhD in 2014.'

What do you see as the influences that have inspired your professional leadership?

'My desire to be a nurse came after a road accident at the age of ten and spending some time in hospital. My decision to be a nurse never changed and I went to university in the 1980s to do one of the very few graduate programmes of its time. My degree at that time also had a focus on social science which has been a hugely influential part of my career. As part of my degree I did social history and social anthropology, so I focused a lot on understanding society and culture, which are pivotal parts of nursing and understanding patient care. In addition it made me see health differently and gain a wide perspective on the role of the nurse and the contribution of nursing to a values-based patient care. I also did politics within my degree, which provided me with a really strong insight into the politics of nursing.

So the social science underpinning was crucial to the shape of my career as a nurse.

I think the first influences on me have been key people – role models. They had stature, knowledge, a presence and wisdom that was appealing. I can think of one of my old lecturers who inspired me. I can still recall her lectures on communication, respect and the value of care – they were awe-inspiring individuals. I think this shaped and influenced my approach to nursing care – I recently bumped into someone who has been one of my students and she related how I had been a role model to her.

Some of the ward sisters I worked with as a staff nurse were also role models as was one of the Directors of Nursing in Lothian then – Mrs Harvey. She was a very "scary" woman but by that I would suggest she commanded total respect and the patients were always at the centre of every conversation she had. She had a presence, a focus on patient care that meant you were clear on what standards she expected from all her nurses.

As my career developed I did find that conferences had quite a key influential impact on my thinking and my career. In particular the RCN International Research Conference allowed me to hear the authors of articles I had read or was reading actually speak – they were normal people with clarity of thought, a voice to the profession. I realised that to be in the research environment I needed to do a PhD – and this led to me doing this. I chose to look at compassionate care as the focus for my thesis which has been a positive motivator in my own career.

It has not just been nurses that have been influential role models to me. Many of my medical colleagues, particularly in haematology, were exemplary role models. I also worked with some really forward-thinking consultants who were pioneers in their field and I learned a huge amount from them – not just in clinical knowledge but also in team work, valuing others and multidisciplinary environments.'

What advice would you provide to student nurses in supporting them to develop their leadership styles and skills?

'Get involved: as a student get involved with things in the clinical environment such as audit or research. Think out of the box and get involved in opportunities you normally wouldn't have the chance to. Don't be afraid to stick your head above the parapet and get yourself noticed.

Education is a key part of developing your leadership skills – lifelong learning whether in a subject, clinical environment or because of the people you meet in an educational environment.

Never compromise your own values base – in order to do this you really do have to understand your own values base, know it, believe in it and stick with it.

Recognise when you do need support – and where that support is going to come from. Recognising times when you need support is pivotal to your own development.'

· ·

VIGNETTE 10.5

Dr Colette Ferguson, Director of Nursing, Midwifery and Allied Health Professions: NHS Education Scotland

Career trajectory

'I began my career in nursing at the age of 17 years. It wasn't something I had planned or considered well in advance as I had no family members who had been in nursing and I knew little about it. On leaving school I undertook a two year enrolled nurse programme not really appreciating the different programmes available.

From day one I enjoyed nursing, particularly my early experiences in care of the elderly. After one year as an enrolled nurse I knew this was the career for me and I decided to commence my RGN training. At this time there were no bridging courses and it meant starting from the beginning and undertaking a three year programme. I enjoyed the learning and the greater understanding of my patients' conditions and the nursing interventions.

I worked as staff nurse for a short time in a general medical ward and then went on to become a registered mental health nurse (RMN) – which again I really enjoyed, and it proved to be one of the most valuable learning experiences which informed my clinical practice thereafter. I would have considered specialising in mental health when an opportunity to work in Gibraltar came my way. I further developed my knowledge, skill and experience working as a senior staff nurse in a medical ward in Gibraltar. Working with patients and staff in a different country and from a different culture was a fantastic experience.

I returned to Scotland for personal reasons and worked as a district nurse for a short period before taking up my first post as a ward sister. Being a ward sister was one of the most rewarding jobs of my career. Leading a ward team and caring for patients and families often under difficult circumstances was both challenging and rewarding. Developing strong relationships across the multi-professional team was essential.

As a ward sister I was aware of the limited opportunities for personal development. Seeing skilled nurses having to leave practice for career development in education or management left me quite frustrated. This was a turning point in my career. I decided to become a clinical teacher so that I could develop my own knowledge but also keep my direct clinical care role. I worked as a clinical teacher for about three years before (reluctantly) undertaking the nurse tutors' course and becoming a lecturer.

In the early 1990s I undertook a full time master's degree at the University of Edinburgh, with my dissertation focusing on student support in practice. On return to my post I played a key role in designing and implementing a mentorship and support system for student nurses for their practice learning experience. I was then lucky enough to build on this experience through my PhD study of the student experience of preceptorship and learning in practice.

In 2003 I commenced work with NHS Education for Scotland (NES), which had only been established a year earlier. My portfolio included national strategic leadership for practice learning and in particular I was instrumental in establishing the Practice Education Facilitator (PEF) role and building the practice education infrastructure for nurses and midwives in Scotland. In NES I have used the findings of my PhD not only to introduce the PEF role in nursing but into wider practice across the country and also across other professions.

My strong focus on supporting learning in practice to ensure the best outcomes for patients continues to drive my ambitions. In NES this informed my leadership while Programme Director, Associate Director and now Director of Nursing, Midwifery and Allied Health Professions.'

What do you see as the influences that have inspired your professional leadership?

'One person early on in my career who really pushed me was my course leader. I think he recognised my potential when I was a student nurse and later he encouraged me to do my master's degree and my PhD, something I would not have considered without this encouragement.

I wouldn't say he was a role model but he was a challenger – he pushed me – encouraged me and recognised the potential that I probably didn't see in myself.

Another influence was a very strong ward sister whom I saw as a clinical role model, her focus was always on ensuring each patient's care was to the highest quality and I've never forgotten the way in which she shared her knowledge and skill and the impact this had on my learning.

Another was the frustration as a ward sister knowing that skilled nurses were leaving for career opportunities away from patient care. The educational opportunities were not really available and I passionately believed in education and the need to keep up to date and to have a system that was fair, transparent and supportive. This was a very strong influence on my focus on practice-based learning while doing my master's degree and my PhD. This is also echoed in my pursuit of a stronger focus and approach to clinical academic careers – the importance of the relationship between education, research and practice for the continuing improvement in patient care and experience is pivotal.'

What advice would you provide to student nurses in supporting them to develop their leadership styles and skills?

'First and foremost, don't forget that our primary purpose is to provide the highest quality care and experience to patients … that's what it is all about!

Keep a focus on the outcomes you are trying to achieve.

Understand the Code and what it means in your leadership journey.

Honesty and integrity as a leader are essential.

Recognising yourself, your own strengths and limitations, is key to leadership development.

Seek feedback and use it well to help you move forward and improve.

Recognise and grasp opportunities – sometimes you can let things go but taking opportunities is vital.

Recognise strong positive role models and consider what you can learn from them.

I still think of patients I have looked after and I know I made a difference to their day or their life – this has been a focus and driver in all that I do.

Being a nurse is a privileged position and it's important for students and all nurses to really appreciate and value this.'

· ·

VIGNETTE 10.6

Professor Tracy Humphrey, Dean of the School of Health & Social Care, Edinburgh Napier University

Career trajectory

'My pre-registration education was in a small university campus in the North of Scotland in the late 1990s at diploma level. I knew that I had to, and wanted to, extend my experiences beyond a district general hospital and rural community, so when I graduated I moved to the North East of Scotland to work in a large tertiary maternity unit. Due to the scale and remit of the unit, I knew I would have the opportunity to gain skills in areas such as high dependency care for women, intensive care for neonates, specialist obstetric services, pregnancy loss. My ambition at that point was to return after a few years and be a community midwife in a rural area and later in my career progress to being a team leader. That felt quite stretching at the time and I thought it would take me most of my career to achieve it. I knew that continuing my education was an essential part of achieving my career aspirations, so I worked full time and studied part time to do my degree. I wanted to learn and develop my thinking more, and to be honest I really enjoyed it.

I finished my degree and then went on to undertake a master's degree. Again, I didn't discuss this with anyone at work, as there were no role models. None of the midwives that worked clinically had an MSc. The only midwives I knew that did, worked in the research centre in the hospital which was part of the university or taught at the university. I didn't aspire to be a research midwife or an educator, I just enjoyed being challenged and learning new knowledge and skills. I applied and was promoted to a 'junior sister' as it was at that time. I was based in the midwife-led intrapartum unit and was among a team of eight midwives who were responsible for leading that service. I really thrived in that role, it was my first experience of being, what I thought at the time, a leader. I was more autonomous, able to influence service development and practice more and could use my education to inform others' practice, not just my own. I did this for two and a half years before being promoted to a sister in a busy labour ward. About two years into the job I saw an advert for a research training scheme which at the time was being supported by the Scottish Government, NHS Education Scotland and the Health Foundation. At that time midwives with PhDs weren't really heard of and so unsurprisingly there was not a lot of support from my midwifery and obstetric colleagues. However, I did apply because I was quite frustrated by a clinical issue, which was about the lack of informed consent for induction of labour and women's poor experiences of care. I saw this as an opportunity to do research that could inform practice and improve women's care. That is what motivated me the most, not the opportunity to do a PhD. I applied and was the only midwife awarded a studentship or fellowship. In order to demonstrate my commitment to clinical practice, I continued to work one day per week in practice throughout my studentship (three years). I was embedded within a multidisciplinary research team within a medical school and this allowed me to get involved in other related health services research projects. During my studentship I started to support these projects by helping with data collection, then analysis, then grant proposals, and by the time I graduated I was a co-applicant on externally funded research. This gave me "research training" while I was doing my PhD, which has been invaluable since.

I completed my PhD in three years and applied for a consultant midwife position in the North East of Scotland. I was successful and did this role for over three years. This was a dream job as I was 50% in clinical practice, developing innovative midwife-led care, leading service delivery and practice. I also had an education, research and policy role. It gave me a national profile in Scotland and the UK and I became a government advisor for maternal and newborn policy. I was also an Honorary Research Fellow at the University of Aberdeen in the Department of Obstetrics and Gynaecology. During this time I also became a Visiting Professor at the School of Nursing and Midwifery, Robert Gordon University.

In 2012, I was appointed to a Clinical Professor of Midwifery role which was a joint appointment between the university and the NHS. My role in both organisations was aligned to providing strategic leadership in relation to maternity services/midwifery, service innovation and evaluation and clinical leadership in a system-wide review of maternity services. Within the university I was the lead for the maternal and child health academic development group: this included programme delivery, research/scholarship and commercialisation.

Then in 2015, I moved into my current role as Dean of Nursing, Midwifery and Social Care. Leading one of the largest schools of nursing and midwifery in the UK.'

What do you see as the influences that have inspired your professional leadership?

'My first inspiration in relation to professional leadership was in my pre-registration education. It was in the Highland Campus of the University of Stirling and therefore we were educated by a small midwifery education team, comprised of only two lecturers. This was my first exposure to "role models" and both of our lecturers were credible. They had authentic experience as midwives both nationally and internationally and used this in the classroom to teach, which brought the subject alive for me. They were respected within the clinical community and had insights and importantly opinions about contemporary midwifery practice and policy which they willingly shared and discussed with us. Their passion was infectious and you could tell that they genuinely cared about us as students and this propelled me to do well as I wanted to make them proud.

Since then, I have had four informal and formal mentors/role models in my career, and that is what has mainly inspired my professional leadership. For me they have been credible, knowledgeable and displayed consistent behaviours, they are visionary, self-motivated, hard-working and committed. They have also been compassionate, fair and empathetic to others. They have inspired me to be who I have become and they have also been the ones to notice what my potential is as I have never been very good at that. I have tried to emulate their approach to leadership whilst being authentic to myself.

If I am honest, and I think this is less relevant now, but I have been inspired in my own professional leadership by others who are not good role models, i.e. I have learned how to lead by knowing that I have to do it differently and better than others around me.

Until recently, I haven't found leadership programmes that are specifically for nursing or midwifery particularly insightful as I think they are often artificial and navel gazing. However, I cannot say that about the Florence Nightingale Scholarship that I have secured. Probably as it has used examples from industry, arts and drama, and other areas or professionals that we can learn a lot from. It also has a bespoke element, so you can tailor it towards your own needs which is more relevant at this stage of my career I think, rather than more generic courses/programmes.

Ultimately, what has inspired my own professional leadership is to improve patient care and experiences. That is what motivates me the most, it sounds corny but it really is so, as they are ultimately why we are here doing what we do. It isn't about the profession – that is secondary to improving health.'

What advice would you provide to student nurses in supporting them to develop their leadership styles and skills?

'Pay attention to the "leaders" around you and reflect on how their behaviour affects others either positively or otherwise and learn from them.

One size doesn't fit all – you will not find one style that works in all situations or with everyone. You need to adapt depending on what and who you are leading.

Read about leadership theories beyond nursing and midwifery, as there is a lot to learn from other professions and disciplines.

Self-reflection is essential, as it is essential for the development of your leadership skills.

Don't be scared to ask for feedback as this will enhance your skills.

Consider, but not over-analytically, how your behaviour may be interpreted by others.'

Activity 11.1

Having read the narratives from the six leaders introduced in this book take a moment to consider the following:

- What key issues are emerging from these leaders' stories for you?
- How important do you think role models have been to you in your career so far?
- What aspects of their advice have most resonance with you?

KEY POINTS FROM THE LEADERSHIP NARRATIVES

Two key and strong themes were identified from the leadership narratives: role models and professional leadership.

Role models

A number of the leaders interviewed were able to point to *role models* as a key influence and impact on their own careers. In particular, the impact of their professional leadership as role models was noted within these narratives. Fowler (2012) identifies the importance of role models and the influence they can have on staff by the transference of their knowledge to practice. A number of other authors have recognised the importance of role models as a necessary part of career development (Allan et al., 2008; Gibson, 2004; Cleary et al., 2013). Role models as leaders are of course not just important for student nurses or newly qualified nurses but also continue to be an important influence on the profession as a whole. Anionwu (2009) demonstrates this by recognising the importance of nursing leaders across the globe in raising their voice on difficult policy issues.

Professional leadership

It could be argued that role models also provide *professional leadership*. Macleod Clark (2014: 98) suggests that the nursing profession in recent years has suffered from a lack of identifiable professional leadership:

> The persistent emphasis on organisational change has been to the detriment of professional vision and has almost certainly inhibited the development of robust pathways which produce strong leaders in clinical practice.

Whilst she argues this in the context of clinical academic research and leadership, the pivotal point of her argument is around the need for strong nursing leaders to have a 'professional vision' – a voice that the nursing profession can identify with, that stands up for patient care, nursing policy and the advancement of the profession of nursing as a whole. Freshwater (2014) in the same journal also suggests that professional leadership is essential to deal with the constant issues of change in healthcare, which is an inevitable aspect of global health.

SUMMARY

There is much we can learn from listening to the voices of others. This chapter has uniquely provided an opportunity to listen and learn from those who have advanced their careers. Their advice is given in a manner that allows you to consider its relevance to your own career, personality, strengths, weaknesses and leadership style. They act as role models for the profession, which the literature identifies as having a key impact on our thinking. Finally, they offer a 'professional' voice, a voice that at its heart has the progression and advancement of nursing

FURTHER RESOURCES

Wangensteen, S., Johansson, I.S. and Nordström, G. (2008) 'The first year as a graduate nurse – an experience of growth and development'. *Journal of Clinical Nursing*, 17(14): 1877–85.

To access further resources related to this chapter, please visit the companion website at https://study.sagepub.com/taylor

REFERENCES

Allan, H.T., Smith, P.A. and Lorentzon, M. (2008) 'Leadership for learning: a literature study of leadership for learning in clinical practice'. *Journal of Nursing Management*, 16(5): 545–55.

Anionwu. E. (2009) 'Strong nursing leaders are role models for students'. *Nursing Standard*, 23(51): 26.

Cleary, M., Horsfall, J. and Jackson, D. (2013) 'Role models in mental health nursing: the good, the bad and the possible'. *Issues in Mental Health Nursing*, 34: 635–6.

Fowler, J. (2012) 'Professional development: from staff nurse to nurse consultant. Part 6: Importance of role models'. *British Journal of Nursing*, 21(5): 311.

Freshwater, D. (2014) 'Board editorial: The challenge of global leadership: managing change, leading movement'. *Journal of Research in Nursing*, 19(2): 93–7.

Gibson, D.E. (2004) 'Role models in career development: new directions for theory and research'. *Journal of Vocational Behavior*, 65(1): 134–56.

Macleod Clark, J. (2014) 'Guest editorial: Clinical academic leadership – moving the profession forward'. *Journal of Research in Nursing*, 19(2): 98–101.

11 THE STUDENT NURSE AS LEADER

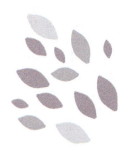

Ruth Taylor

With thanks to Amy Tran, Carol Roughley, Emma Wolton, Louisa McGee, Clare Benney, Hannah Leggett, Lorraine Thompsett, Briannie Falconer, Laura Berrill – all students at Anglia Ruskin University.

Visit the companion website at https://study.sagepub.com/taylor to watch some students interviews

Chapter learning outcomes

On completion of this chapter you will be able to:

- Appreciate the scope of the student nurse as a developing leader.
- Map out your own leadership experiences and aspirations – past, present and future.
- Pinpoint your inspirations and contributions so that you can clarify the way in which you, as a student nurse, can achieve your potential as a leader.

Key concepts

Student nurse, leadership, leader

INTRODUCTION

The purpose of this chapter is to bring to life the ways in which you as a student nurse are, or can be, a leader as you progress through your course and on to the point at which you qualify as a nurse. As you will have gathered, we (Brian and I) believe that student nurses are developing leaders in their own right and we want to inspire you to fulfil your full potential as a leader. As you will have seen if you have worked your way through this book (or dipped in and out of it depending on your approach), all the authors have focused on the student nurse as a developing leader – with examples offered of ways that you can expand your leadership skills throughout. What this chapter provides is examples of *real* people's voices – student nurses who have had varied experiences and have articulated the ways in which they feel they are (or aren't) leaders, and what they see as 'good' leadership. To do this, I interviewed nine student nurses. Whilst I felt that I could have done this without ethical approval, I sought approval from my university research ethics panel so that I could ensure that I conducted myself in an ethical manner within the context of writing this chapter and in future publications. A purposive sample of students was recruited via email. The email explained the project so that the students were clear about the focus and they were provided with an information sheet and consent form. The students were asked to contact me directly with notes of interest. I was delighted by the response, and contacted all of those who got in touch with me, resulting in the nine interviews. Semi-structured interviews were undertaken. They were audio recorded and transcribed. The purpose of the interviews was to:

- Explore experiences and key moments of leadership learning, inspiration and impact.
- Explore their views on the student nurse as leader.

The interviews were then used to develop the vignettes that you see within this chapter. Each of the vignettes touches only a small part of what these students said to me. The vignettes aim to illustrate the aspects of leadership that seemed to be of most importance to the students at the time, and to link to some of what is discussed within the chapters in this book. Just so you know, the vignettes were sent to each of the students so that they could let me know if they disagreed with anything that I had written. All of them agreed to me using their names – I see this chapter as a joint effort and they are therefore credited as co-authors of this chapter.

I hope that what you read here is inspiring and insightful for your own learning. It has been both of these things for me – I knew that our student nurses were amazing people, but when I listened to what they were telling me, I felt humbled by their commitment to our profession, and clear that nursing lies in the hands of practitioners who are making a positive difference to those people they come into contact with. Thank you to each and every one of these students. So, without further ado, I move into the main part of this chapter.

STUDENT VOICES: VIGNETTES OF LEADERSHIP LEARNING, INSPIRATION AND IMPACT

Each of the vignettes offers perspectives on various aspects of leadership – what each person sees as 'good' leadership and a personal example (a view of an inspirational leader, a situation in which they have demonstrated leadership, or an issue that they see as hugely important for the leadership of nursing). The details that I provide here were the situation at the time that I did the interviews. I didn't ask much in the way of demographic details – just a couple of things so that you have some details. The vignettes are presented in modified versions of their own words – some quotes are used but by necessity abridged with the aim of conveying the essence of their views. I am not claiming that these interviews are representative of all students' views or in any way representative as a sample in terms of demographics or field of practice. I simply interviewed those individuals who got back to me after being approached to be part of the project.

Activities

For each of the vignettes, you could jot down words or phrases that resonate with you and the kind of leader that you want to be.

You can also identify what aspects of the leadership theory these vignettes refer to. For example, do any of the students identify particular traits or behaviours in the leaders that they describe?

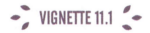

VIGNETTE 11.1

Amy Tran – Calm during the storm

Amy's field of practice is children's and young people's nursing, she is a third year student nurse, and 20 years old. Amy had worked in children's nurseries prior to starting her course.

'A leader is someone who takes control of the situation, ensuring that everyone knows what's going on. The main things for me are control and structure in leadership. What's also important is that the leader is someone who is good at communicating, has the trust and respect of others. It's not hierarchy – it's more about being able to trust the leader's knowledge and competency and trusting the leader as a person (rather than "oh you're higher than me, I should listen to you"). A leader also has to have faith in their own self and has to feel confident in what they are doing. I feel that you have to believe in yourself before others can believe in you. Being calm is also important. A nurse who was holding the bleep one day was so inspirational to me. Her demeanour was so calm and the way she dealt with people was calm as well. We had anxious parents and the way she communicated with them was so calming – her body language, the way she kept order was impressive, and just how she spoke to everyone. I'm just impressed that people can deal with situations that are way over their heads or have been given more than they can handle – but they can still manage it, can still be calm and collected! They make the whole environment calmer, not calm *before* the storm; calm *during* the storm.

Relationships are the key because once you've built that relationship with your staff, with the patients, with the patients' parents ... you've built that trust. An example of when I did this was when I was leading parents towards aiding their child to better health – if that makes sense. On this one occasion, I spoke to the parents alone explaining what the procedure would be and that I would be there to distract their child, getting the bubbles out which is always fun! I had the chance to build a rapport in a very short space of time, and me being in the room made it a lot easier for the parents and for the child. Having the parents tell me a bit about their child helped me to build trust and aided me to distract the child. Parents know best!'

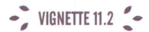

VIGNETTE 11.2

Carol Roughley – Standing up and having a voice

Carol is 48 years old, a third year student nurse in the adult field, and had previously volunteered at a hospital.

'A nursing leader is someone who has the ability to keep the whole team of healthcare professionals working well together, someone who is approachable and who respects everyone whatever they are doing – whether they are the domestic or the senior consultant. I'm working with someone like that at the moment – she's absolutely incredible. Anyone who talks about her, talks about her with so much admiration. She is loved by everybody. She's really professional, she's caring, she loves having students. I went onto her ward and said that I was starting placement in a few days' time. She was actually quite busy but she said come into my office for a few minutes and she was just lovely. She said, "We are so looking forward to having you here". She really makes the students feel welcome on her ward. She's an incredible nurse and person. She just gets it right. There was a situation where a relative was really angry about a situation. She did nothing except sit and listen to the patient and his daughter, she didn't say a word and wasn't defensive. She just apologised and said that she would do everything within her means to make sure that the situation never happened again. They felt listened to and like we cared. For me, leadership is about how you decide to practice.

Thinking about how students can make a difference as leaders in practice – I do believe that student nurses can make a difference but there are times when we can be diplomatically silenced. It's about purely being able to voice your opinion and say that this is not OK. And when you're told [by a member of staff] to know when it's not your battle, just keep quiet and get on with it ... I don't like that approach and I don't think it's necessary to have that approach. How sad that people who are actually willing to stand up for good care and get the best for their patients, are actually perceived as almost trouble causers. People need to feel that they are listened to. I am so serious about making sure that people do take patients' experiences and needs seriously. If you haven't got time to hold my hand or put your hand on someone's shoulder ... It doesn't take anything, to be honest – just care!

I attended the Royal College of Nursing Congress last year in Bournemouth. I got to stand up in front of a hundred students and there were a few nurses there. And at the end of it they came up to me and said "because of you I'm now going to say something if I see anything", and I thought wow – that's great!'

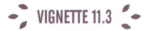

VIGNETTE 11.3

Emma Wolton – Transition

Emma has recently qualified as a children's and young people's nurse (she did the students' thanks address at graduation on behalf of her peers!), is 29, and worked as an au pair before starting her course.

'I would say that leadership is being at the helm of a good team, a successful team. Keeping staff morale high is an important part of being a good leader but there are definitely different styles of leadership and I suppose it's about fitting that personality to that style of leadership and making it work. I think that the leader is normally the person who organises the team, who takes the leading role. But I think that there are role models as well who can demonstrate good practice and share that amongst the other team members. When I was in one of my placements as a student nurse, there was a very good mentor who kind of took it upon himself to be a leader of student nurses and would lead teaching sessions for us. He was an excellent speaker and obviously very experienced and knew his stuff. He was friendly and kind, and well respected amongst the team. I think that being very knowledgeable and having that experience meant that he was trusted. He was also very good with the patients, having a good rapport, and he was funny with them as well. He was able to calm people down especially in serious situations, making people feel at ease so that they felt confident in their own abilities and didn't need to be stressed or frantic. This nurse that I'm talking about was inspiring the next generation of nurses, leading the way for what would shape the department in years to come, and I think inspiring nurses to want to learn.

When I was a student nurse, I didn't feel like I acted like a leader but there were a couple of times when staff nurses remarked that student nurses are the ones who have access to the current information and legislation through journal articles and other information. I do think that when there are things that are slightly amiss in a placement, then it would be the student nurse who leads how they deal with that situation – if poor care or uncompassionate care is going on. The student nurse can act in an appropriate way and not normalise the working culture. But I was lucky that I didn't come across anything like that – the nursing was all really good.

Now that I'm qualified I feel a responsibility for the students as I am in charge of how they might practise in the future when I am working with them. I personally found the transition to being a newly qualified nurse quite difficult as my final placement was in the community and I didn't have the opportunity to delegate for example. I still think it's a jump for everyone because you have all that extra responsibility. You become the leader of that patient's care and there is a lot of responsibility in that. I am enjoying my rotation and am interested to see how I find my next placement which is in elective care and outpatients. I could see myself working there or perhaps as a community nurse. I'll hopefully work up the scale and at some point do a master's. I'd like to be a sister in the future.'

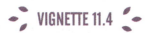

VIGNETTE 11.4

Louisa McGee – Leading other students

Louisa is a third year student nurse in children's and young people's nursing, she is 25 years old, and worked as a healthcare assistant when she left school – mainly in adult settings.

Watch Louisa's interview on the companion website at https://study.sagepub.com/taylor

'To me, a leader is someone that you can turn to for guidance if you need it; someone who steers you rather than lectures and stands over you; someone you can turn to if you need help and can support your learning and facilitate it. I've found someone on every placement who I could turn to if I needed help, someone who trusted me and didn't feel like it was an inconvenience if I asked them a stupid question (or what you may feel is a stupid question). Once I've found that person I tend to stick with them! This way of working with students makes me feel really good because I've done things by using my own initiative.

On a busy day in one of my placements, some of the patients were really anxious and it was rubbing off on everyone with one patient being a bit aggressive. The sister dealt with it really well. She didn't say anything that other people hadn't said before, but she just managed to calm them all down. She was direct but nice about it. Having someone who appears calm, whether she is calm or not, just really helps.

Now that third year has come along, I do find that first and second year students are looking at you as a leader because I did it in first year as a student. I remember being terrified and know how these students feel. I feel that I have to set an example. You just have to reassure them. I do like the leadership part of it and there's something nice about being able to help them in a professional way. I remember that myself, and that situation where you think that you'll never know as much as the third years. And now that I'm here, I'm starting to realise how much I have learnt! I've been a student rep for three years now. We've got a Facebook group which is really handy for sharing information and keeping people in touch when we are in placements. Sometimes things crop up and I ask the other students if they want me to raise them with the university.'

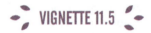

VIGNETTE 11.5

Clare Benney – Learning through example, not hierarchy

Clare is 27 years old, and in the second year of her adult nursing course. She had not had 'official' caring experience but had looked after her granddad palliatively. She had also volunteered in Cambodia in a medical centre. She had done a degree in English and History before deciding to become a nurse.

'I think that leadership in nursing practice is probably different from generic leadership and it requires a certain expertise. You need the knowledge-base to lead and an absolute array of communicative and personal skills. You have to be sensitive, compassionate and hard working. Where I'm working at the moment is a really acute environment and the leadership doesn't always come from the person in charge. As a student I take leadership from the staff nurses, the healthcare assistants – it isn't always about where you are in the hierarchy, it is who you are as a person.

I've seen inspirational leadership a multitude of times. One that stands out for me is the second cardiac arrest that I ever saw (my first cardiac arrest was mayhem and it really unnerved me as there was no clear leadership). The deputy sister was so calm and very effective; it was fluid as it should be, and she was the entire reason that it was like that because of how she is. Describing what she did will maybe make what I mean clearer. It was visiting time, the patient was unwell but a cardiac arrest was clearly not expected. The patient was talking to her daughter and went into arrest and the daughter screamed out. I went in with the healthcare assistant and just began to pull the bed out as we've been trained to do. Everyone was there within a few seconds but the moment that the deputy sister was there she just stood at the head end of the bed and just calmly in a normal voice said, "Clare, would you please do this", "staff nurse, would you please do that". When the anaesthetist and crash team arrived she still maintained that role and when the resuscitation officer arrived he didn't detract from that, as it was clear that she had it under control. So I think it was her calmness, you could see that she was really at ease with the situation.

Another example was when we were looking after a young woman who was dying. She had a number of children and she was deteriorating rapidly and wanted to be at home. Just by being proactive, the nurse was able to get her home in four hours. She rang everyone – the discharge team, private transport, the district nurses. This doesn't sound like anything outstanding but in a ward as busy as that one it could have been easy to say that there was no time to do what was needed. It was a team effort and I just thought that day, this is how it should be done. If it can be done here, then it can be done elsewhere. The nurse in this ward was a positive role model for me, as was another – both different personalities and approaches (one was very confident and dynamic, direct and an advocate for patients; the other was very quietly spoken and patient). They are very different people but they share the same knowledge-base, patient-centred attitude and can-do approach. They really facilitated my learning.'

- -

❧ VIGNETTE 11.6 ☙

Hannah Leggett – Leading by example

Hannah is coming towards the end of her second year in mental health nursing. She is 33 years old. She had had quite a lot of previous caring experiences, mainly in learning disabilities, having worked in a private company from the age of 17, and then working for an agency in a variety of settings.

'A good leader has organisational skills, makes things work well, and keeps everyone happy. Good leadership needs you to have good relationships with staff and for people to feel happy to do what you need them to do. You have to be open to others' views as well. A leader has to be competent and take responsibility and also motivate people. I also think that leadership is about making the standards and values so it goes from the top down – to lead by example is the easy way to say it. I think that people tend to do a job well when they know the reason that they're doing it rather than just being told that this is what you have to do. If you understand the reason for doing something it makes it more likely that you will do things right and take responsibility for what you're doing. Another thing that I see as important is when the nurse in charge works just as hard as everyone else, having to take on the responsibilities of what only they can do but also taking on any job on a shift. The leader should also be supportive. In this same placement, there was a problem and the nurse that I've spoken about was supportive of the rest of the team, spoke about the issues and the process of what was going to happen. So rather than not talking about it, she recognised there was a problem and that people were upset about it and made sure that people felt supported. She would speak out for staff, for example if staffing levels were too low, and she understood that people had to work harder. She was fair and competent and people trusted her. She also built good relationships with patients and was friendly and happy. She led by example!

I learnt a lot from her and now I feel that I wouldn't ask anyone to do something that I wouldn't do myself. I would let people know why I was asking them to do something, not just say it is a policy. One example of where you might say that I showed leadership was when I was on a ward where there was a high-spirited lady. The staff were a bit negative about her but I used to enjoy her company anyway. I gave her quite a lot of my time and I did notice that other people started to see her in a different way. I think I raised her profile, you know, people's opinions of her. I think the healthcare assistants saw the standard of someone else and they appreciated that, and it made a difference to some of what they did – small things like making sure someone had their hearing aid in their ear. I suppose as a student nurse you are supernumerary and have more time so you sort of *see* the issues.'

• •

❧ VIGNETTE 11.7 ❧

Lorraine Thompsett – Changing and challenging practice

Lorraine is a second year nurse, almost ready to go into her third year of an adult nursing course. She is 44 years old. She had trained as a phlebotomist, then as an assistant practitioner in mammography.

'Nursing leadership is probably setting an example to the people around you. So not necessarily hierarchy but doing things that maybe challenge what's already going on and showing a different perspective of practice. A leader is also proactive in doing things and teaching people, sharing experiences; challenging practice and setting a good example so that people will follow you if they feel that your practice is perhaps better than what they already know.

My last mentor was quite an inspiration. I would like to be like her. On that ward, they had just taken on team nursing rather than individual nursing which wasn't very well accepted among the team, and she didn't agree with the change either. She was a senior staff nurse, not management but she spoke to everyone, told them her view but said that they would have to get on with it. She devised a plan, made a spreadsheet and brought people together hourly to communicate and for a bit of a debrief. This made it easier for everyone to work, as they were struggling with the team nursing. She was assertive, and put across the view that they were a team who had to look after the patients. She was seen as part of the team. She listened to people, was approachable and had a knack of telling people what needed to be done without offending them. She was just very calm.

I have challenged and changed practice in a placement. I questioned what they were doing in the particular placement and asked why they were doing it that way. People responded by saying "because we've been told to". One example was to do with the way they went about giving residents their breakfast. I decided to take the head of the trolley and the healthcare assistant followed me. I woke the residents up gently and asked them what they wanted, trying to promote choice. I was approaching the residents in a different way from what they had been used to. In this situation I had to approach the university about what was going on.

As a third year, I realise that I have grown as a person and become more confident because knowledge gives you confidence. I think for me as an individual I don't feel like I've progressed massively until something happens like taking a first year under my wing and you think, "Wow! I have learnt a lot and do understand a lot of things". I think that students are in a much better position to make change and congratulate where there is good practice.'

• •

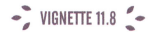

VIGNETTE 11.8

Briannie Falconer – Stepping up

Briannie is 22 years old and in her second year of a children's and young people's nursing course. She was a combat medical technician in the army for two years, and had volunteered at a home for mentally and physically disabled children in South Africa. She had also worked as a carer in the speciality of dementia.

Watch Briannie's interview on the companion website at https://study.sagepub.com/taylor

'I think that leadership in nursing practice can be at any level. It's about showing initiative and a willingness to learn. It's sometimes about stepping up and making the decisions that people don't necessarily want to. So it's not just about being a leader on a good day, but being a leader on a bad day as well.

I saw the sister on the ward I was on as an inspirational leader. One day she got a phone call from a very distressed mum saying "I know I was supposed to bring my child in for surgery today but I turned my back and he took a mouthful of his brother's cereal". The sister could very easily have stopped the child coming in for surgery but she said that she would speak to the team and see what they could do. She went out of her way to get hold of the team and moved the child up the theatre list so that he could come in for his surgery. She went above and beyond – she had other things that she needed to be doing that morning but she put them on hold. She was a champion for that child and a good example for the nurses on that ward – this is what you should be trying to do for every patient. She was a role model in the way she approached situations. She wouldn't always take the straightforward route but would look for alternatives. She was calm – she always said that there was no point in panicking about things because it's not going to fix anything, no point in getting stressed! She was never imposing and was the first one to get involved, the first one to step up. She said to me that I shouldn't underestimate the impact that I can have as a student nurse. She could see the importance of every person within that setting and that I actually do have a role and responsibility as a student, and that I can impact positively on someone. She made me realise as a first year that I could also step up and be that student who is always asking "can I do that?". You want to look enthusiastic but not pushy, but working with her made me realise that I wasn't being pushy; I was just showing the love of what I was doing.

I think that the minute that you put that uniform on and go out into practice, any patient or family is going to see you as a leader because you've got a uniform on.'

· ·

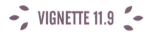

VIGNETTE 11.9

Laura Berrill – Caring in leadership

Laura is a 21 year old student nurse in children's and young people's nursing, who had worked as a play leader before coming into nursing. She is in the third year of her course.

'I think that leadership is something that we all do at some point no matter what level we are – whether it's a second year helping out a first year or a ward manager looking after their team. It's just part of caring for each other as staff I suppose. In terms of the management role there are obviously further leadership skills that you need: communication skills and management skills rather than leadership skills. But it's something that anyone and everyone can do if it's something that they want to do. I think that you can lead without realising you're leading. I've been in situations where I've just shown people how to do something for the first time, or just saying to them "it's alright, everyone was new once". You're helping them and leading them but not saying "I'm above you". I think that teaching others is very much a leadership role that students take on.

I can't stand it when managers sit in an office and tell people what to do and don't do any of it themselves. They tell you what to do but they actually have no idea what it feels like to do some of those things. So to have someone who will support you, just behind you, knowing that they will muck in – I really appreciate that in nursing leadership. Leadership is also about giving a caring professional response to someone when they are having personal difficulties, and being honest with you about how well you are doing as a student.

I love having students with me on placement and getting the chance to teach them. I feel confident, and am quite calm. I can be thrown in at the deep end and just take a deep breath and get on with it! I've come across great nurses and mentors who could empathise with what it's like to be a student in particular situations.'

. . . .

MOLLY CASE

Finally, I want to write a bit about Molly Case. Molly Case is a nurse, a poet, and a spoken word artist. Some of you may be familiar with Molly as she came to the fore in 2013 at the RCN Congress where she performed one of her poems 'Nursing the Nation'. At that time she was a student nurse. The poem's words resonated with thousands of nurses across our nation at a time when there was a great deal of media attention which focused on caring, or the perceived lack of it. The narrative associated with this media coverage sometimes pointed to nursing students as being 'at fault', something that Molly addressed in her poem. Here is the link at which you can see and hear her perform: www.youtube.com/watch?v=XOCda6OiYpg. Molly clearly articulates the passion, motivation and expertise of student nurses as they go about doing extraordinary things on what seem like ordinary days to you as nurses. She has gone on to be named in the *Health Service Journal*'s Inspirational Women's list. I am not saying that you will all go on to do things that are recognised in this way at a national level – though some of you will I am sure. What I am saying is that you all have a voice and, as some of the student nurses in this chapter show, you can use it to really make a difference.

NURSING THE NATION

A woman comes in,
too young to bear this;
she's got a disease that will make her miss –
her daughter's wedding day,
her first grandchild being born.
How would that feel, to have that all torn
away from you?

I can't answer that question,
it's not my place to say,
but I can tell you what we did for her,
how we helped her get through the day.
A cup of tea there and one for all her family,
as they came, throughout the night,
what a sight; there were loads of them.
To help her fight the awful pain of it,
paying last visits, we wouldn't let them miss it –
farewell from a brother,
last kisses with their mother –
holiest love, love like no other.

Maybe there's bad ones,
no doubt that there are,
but for this list I'm writing
we don't want the same tar-brush,
crushing our careers before they've even started;
how could you say this
about people so big-hearted?

Who would have thought we'd be having to
    defend?
We don't do this for our families,
we don't do this for our friends,
but for strangers.
Because this is our vocation
and we're sick and tired
of being told we don't do enough for this nation.
So listen to us, hear us goddamn roar;
you say we're not doing enough?
Then we promise we'll do more.
This time, next time,
there's nothing we can't handle,
even if you bring us down,
show us scandal, scandal, scandal.

You remember that man covered in burns head
    to toe?
I don't think you do
'cause you were on that TV show:
lipgloss-kissed women on daytime TV,
come into our world, see things that we see.

One lady, passing, had no relatives to stay.
We sang her to sleep, let angels take her away.
Were you there that day when we held her
    hand?
Told her nothing would harm her,
that there was a higher plan.
Saw her face as she remembered a faith she'd
    once held,
watched her breath in the room as she finally
    exhaled.

Why don't you meet us? Come, shake our hands.
Try to fit it in between having tea with
    your fans.
Your hands are so soft and mine are cracked.
Why don't you let us on air?
Let us air the facts.

We've washed and shrouded people
that we've never known,
pinned flowers to the sheet
and told them they're still not alone.
Shown families to the faith room
and watched them mourn their dead,
then got back to work, bathed patients, made
    beds.

Hindus, Muslims, Jews and Sikhs,
Buddhists and Christians and just people off the
    street,
we've cared for them all and we love what
    we do,
we don't want a medal, we just want to show
    you.
So listen to us, hear us goddamn roar;
you say we're not doing enough?
Then we promise we'll do more.

Activity 11.2

Based on these vignettes, the story of Molly and your own experiences, you might like to now draw up a blueprint for leadership – one that you aspire to and will always work towards in the many situations and contexts that you will find yourself in as you continue your career in nursing. I'd suggest something short and snappy – something that you can pin to your desk or fridge to remind yourself that this is the kind of leader you are or want to be:

'This is the kind of leader I am, or that I aspire to be ...'

SUMMARY

The learning from this chapter is for you to determine. I am sure that it will be very personal and will be based on your own experiences and your reflections on how these voices resonated, or otherwise, with your own views. Hopefully, you will have seen something here that inspires you and will enable you to continue your growth as a leader.

Some key learning points from this chapter include:

- Trust, caring, approachability, respect, interest in others, person- and patient-focused are some of the characteristics that are important for good leadership.
- Excellent communication skills are crucial to the development of relationships and the ability of someone to lead a team.
- Calmness is an attribute for leaders to encompass within their practice so that others feel able to tackle challenging situations when they occur.

EPILOGUE

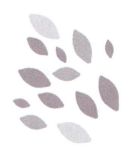

Personal reflections

Brian Webster-Henderson and Ruth Taylor

Visit the companion website at https://study.sagepub.com/taylor to watch Ruth and Brian's interviews.

It should come as no surprise that in writing a book about leadership and in encouraging you as readers through many of the activities within this book to 'reflect', we as editors and authors have been motivated to reflect on our own careers and leadership journeys. In doing so we have been identifying, analysing and reflecting on pivotal aspects of our careers, individuals we have met, worked with, learned from and respected. What follows are our own personal reflections of our leadership journeys within our nursing careers in the hope that you might learn from our reflections and consider and refine your developing leadership skills.

RUTH'S REFLECTIONS ON HER LEADERSHIP JOURNEY

I want to tell you a bit about my leadership journey. In my reflection, I share some personal things – nothing too deep but enough so that you can see that my leadership journey is inextricably entwined with my personal life and circumstances. I do not hold myself up as someone special; but offer up my story as a way of showing how I learned and developed myself.

Of profound importance to my decision to become a nurse were some decisions that my parents made when I was young. I moved secondary schools three times and the last move meant that I had to move from England to Scotland (a country that I now love very much). What this meant for me was that I couldn't undertake the appropriate language qualifications at school that would have enabled me to go to university to do what I had planned – having studied three languages plus two lots of English at O level I'd set my sights on a career as a translator. I changed education systems and arrived at a school where the careers teacher saw nursing or secretarial work as the only opportunities for young women. I chose nursing – which meant I could leave school and get on with life. I did my nurse training at Addenbrooke's Hospital in Cambridge in the 1980s and finally found my 'place' in nursing when I worked on the oncology ward in my final placement. I knew that this was where I belonged and continued to work in that area for most of my clinical career. The sister on that ward, Mary Layton, was a role model for me – she was the first nurse leader that I remember really respecting without fear. She wanted the highest quality of care in her ward, and she made sure that we adhered to those high standards. But she was caring, funny, willing to get in and help in any way, and she saw my potential.

I worked in that ward for a few months before packing a rucksack and setting off for Australia via Indonesia and Singapore. My friend Sarah and I arrived in Sydney with a few hundred pounds in our pockets, worked in a supermarket until our registration came through, and then worked as agency staff nurses in the middle of Sydney. I loved and hated it in equal measure – always terrified about the responsibility that was thrust on me as a newly qualified nurse at the other side of the world. That experience taught me that nurturing people – even staff who are only part of the team for a short period of time – is so important both for that individual and for the people that they are looking after. Sarah and I travelled for a year and then I went back to the UK to do an oncology course at the Royal Marsden Hospital in London. This was when I came across a 'celebrity' nurse – one who had made an impact on our profession. His name was Robert Tiffany. He was a cancer nurse specialist and had written in that area, advocated for that area of specialism, and engaged at a national level. I remember him sweeping into our classroom, all of us in awe of him. In my opinion he raised the profile of nursing, along with some of his contemporaries, and I think I understood then what it meant to be passionate about nursing as a profession.

Life went on. I got married and lived in New Zealand for a while, coming back to the UK again when I was pregnant with my first daughter – the lovely Sophie. I got a job as a staff nurse in the local hospital doing night shifts so that I could juggle being a mum and bringing in some much-needed cash. I enjoyed working there but I am not sure how much the staff enjoyed having me at first. I was concerned about a number of things – just the way things were done, not through any malice but because that's how they did things round there. I spoke up and was supported to make the changes that I had suggested. After a few months I got a job on an oncology ward and decided to sign up for a BSc(Hons) in nursing – my brain needed something to get into and I must have seen that this degree would be essential for me to enhance my career. I had my other lovely daughter, Jo, and not long after that became a single mum. Things got better quickly and I got a second job as a practice nurse. I was learning new skills, developing excellent organisational skills (balancing work and children), and growing in confidence as I continued on my degree. I didn't think of myself as a leader at this time, despite the fact that I was 'in charge' on my night shift job and was working pretty autonomously as a practice nurse.

What I now see as the job that really changed my life came along next – I got a lecturer role at Robert Gordon University. I worked there for 15 years and had a variety of roles working my way up: course leader for a general practice nursing degree, programme leader for the pre-registration nursing course, Associate Head of School, and finally acting Head of School before I set off on a new adventure. The things that impacted on my growth as an academic leader were:

- Learning – I did a master's degree which remains the best educational experience that I have had, opening my mind up to research and helping me to reflect on and understand my potential. I completed a PhD in 2009 and was thrilled to graduate with that.
- I had two wonderful bosses. Jennie Parry was my first Head of School. She taught me lots of things around organisational leadership but mainly believed in me and was an excellent role model. Next was Brian Webster-Henderson – my co-editor – who supported, enabled, critiqued, encouraged, and inspired me (whilst also making me laugh a lot!).
- I was successful in obtaining my professorial title because I had developed a portfolio of teaching, research, policy influence, national and international networks, and publications that all linked up. I had worked out that I needed to find my 'thing' that would make a difference (to students in my case) and that would have high impact. I remember sitting on a train and getting the message that my application for professorship had been accepted, and that was some moment for me.
- The drive that I had to provide for my children – as a single mum with no other income coming in, it was up to me. This external factor was on reflection a pivotal and important aspect in my career, and I was lucky to also have that intrinsic motivation to want to do well and to progress in my career.
- I was fortunate to be awarded a Florence Nightingale Foundation Leadership scholarship which took me all over the world. Probably the most powerful aspects of this experience were a creative leadership retreat in Seattle where I met some amazing female nurse leaders, and the coaching that I continue to engage with.

The things that have motivated me include my children as I've said, and an internal desire to be good at what I do. There are other things as well though. I am an introvert and a woman – these facts impact on me as a leader and I have done lots of work to understand myself and others (especially extroverts!) so that I can carry myself as a leader with confidence (albeit that the confident exterior belies less composed inner feelings sometimes). I have grown to enjoy networking, and understand that I just need to go home to peace and quiet to recharge afterwards!

I am now working as a Pro Vice Chancellor and Dean at Anglia Ruskin University. I went there as Deputy Dean and was appointed to the more senior role a year after I arrived. Again, it is the relationships I have with strong leaders that I feel have enabled me to get to this stage. I have had people see in me what I maybe didn't see in myself and that has given me the confidence to go for the next job. You might have heard about 'imposter syndrome' – this is where people (particularly women) think that they are going to be 'found out', that they are not quite good enough to go for that next promotion, or that they can't see how they got into the position that they have. I admit to sometimes feeling like this, but not as much as I used to. Using coaching, reflecting on my practice, seeing the results of my work and making sure that I tell people about them have led me to believe in myself. As well as these things, it is the fact that I am passionate about the experience of our staff and students, and of course the patients that our students look after, that mean that I am happy to take on a visible leadership role. I want to make a difference.

So, in amongst that story there are some lessons I think:

- Seek out mentors and role models and be willing to have challenging conversations about your skills and attributes.
- Grow your networks – I now have networks right across the globe in Australia, the USA, Malawi and Europe to name a few. Nurture those networks and be generous with your time and contribution to collaborative activities.
- Have reasons to be successful (and success does not equate to promotion; for me it equates to feeling that you are in the right job and are happy) – these will be extrinsic (for me, my children) and intrinsic (the internal drivers that give you passion for what you do).
- Thank people who help you and celebrate others' success. Grasp opportunities – the Florence Nightingale scholarship was life-changing for me but I had to make a decision to just go for it.
- It sounds corny, but tell yourself about the things you are really good at, and congratulate yourself when you do things outside of your comfort zone. And tell other people when you do things well too!
- Nurture others, see their potential and help them find ways to fulfil that potential.
- Keep your eyes on the 'rocks' in your life – these rocks for me are the people that bring me joy: my girls, my husband, family and friends.
- Strive to understand yourself and what makes you tick – for me this was, in part, about understanding what introversion is and realising that it was normal to feel and behave in the way I do (no need for me to be a noisy person, and important for me to appreciate the extroverts).

Some of the things that I am proud of achieving in my career include: the transformation of the student experience at both a local (university) and national level (in Scotland) where I contributed to a wonderful collaboration that led to much change (other authors in this book were part of that too, in particular Mike Sabin); my first academic publication – I wish that I had started earlier; the relationships that I have with the staff I work with and with students; achieving well academically and using the academic work to make a difference in practice; my ability to network in person and through social media.

BRIAN'S REFLECTIONS ON HIS LEADERSHIP JOURNEY

I had never planned on becoming a nurse but had rather set my mind on leaving school, going to university and undertaking a degree in psychology and social administration – with a view to becoming a social worker. I always knew that my mind was truly set on becoming a professional where I was required to support or help individuals. However, in the middle of my then Higher qualifications in Scotland, my mother suddenly died of cancer and my life was turned upside down. I left school having sat only two of the four qualifications I was studying for and immediately started to look after my bereaved father and oldest brother. University was therefore not accessible and over the next few months I looked for alternative routes to become a social worker. As a way of preparing myself for the role, a careers advisor encouraged me to undertake mental health nursing and then go on to do a social work qualification.

During my mental health nurse training at the Sunnyside Royal Hospital in Montrose, I realised that nursing was for me, and in particular I found my passion in supporting those with alcohol and drug misuse problems. I was 20 years and 6 months old when I completed my mental health nurse training and felt incredibly young, naive and inexperienced with life; but I was completely motivated by the dynamic alcohol problems team I worked with – a group of nurses with vast experience who to this day inspire and encourage me to develop my professional career more than they know. The key to working in addictions is around the skills of listening, communication and empowering others with the skills to be self-motivated and succeed. These skills, as a part of my clinical role, have been pivotal to my leadership approach throughout my career: listen – motivate – empower.

For personal reasons I then moved to Portsmouth and worked in an area of mental health that I found less enjoyable, so quickly decided to undertake my adult nurse training. Whilst incredibly rewarding and increasing my clinical knowledge, I was encouraged by a ward sister that I worked with – Brenda Dillon – to go to university (in my spare time) and undertake a degree. She supported my shift patterns and offered financial support to undertake a degree in politics and health administration – which I completed after four years. Not only did this degree enhance my skills of communication and give me a deeper understanding of the politics of the NHS, it also facilitated my ability to stand up for improving patient care and finding innovation, and led to me developing a real hunger to gain a deeper understanding around evidence-based practice.

My career and life events moved me to Southampton where I was a charge nurse in several wards in acute medicine, looking after patients who were seriously acutely ill and supporting staff of all levels of knowledge and abilities to provide the best care they possibly could. It was an exciting time and during this period I undertook a master's degree in advanced healthcare practice – which stretched my thinking to a deeper level and motivated me further to develop my staff to provide evidence-based decision-making in their care provision. I also studied for a postgraduate diploma in education and quickly realised that I wanted to pursue a career in higher education as a way of educating, empowering and motivating others to develop their potential as nurses – at whatever stage.

I became a lecturer at the University of Southampton where I had the privilege of working with a large group of highly motivated, intellectual and practice-focused academics. The School of Nursing and Midwifery was led by Professor Dame Jill Macleod Clark – who remains to this day a hugely influential nurse in terms of policy, regulation, government policy and research. Her skills of challenge and motivation in equal measures, and her ability to see my potential, were key to encouraging me in higher education and in developing a successful career.

I moved to Scotland in 2009 to be Head of the School of Nursing and Midwifery at Robert Gordon University where I met Ruth Taylor – who was my deputy – and together we were able to introduce many innovations for our students with the help and commitment of our academic colleagues. Being a leader in a successful school was nothing compared to being a leader in your *own* school and leading it to continuous success!

My current role at Edinburgh Napier University is as University Dean of Learning and Teaching and a Professor of Nursing. Leadership across a whole organisation such as a university requires many skills that are essential in nursing and that Ruth and I have included in our chapters here – skills of coaching, understanding people and organisations, listening and making choices, taking bold decisions that keep the patient (or in our case the student) at the centre of successful leadership. So in preparing this book my key reflections on leadership in my own life are:

- Sometimes life events – such as bereavement in my case – can provide a platform to learn more about yourself than you know.
- Working with a team of like-minded and equally motivated individuals is a transforming and empowering experience.
- Three key skills as a leader wherever you are: listen – motivate – empower.
- Education is as much around learning about yourself as it is about learning about the subject you are studying for. Through all my degrees, from politics to doctoral studies, I have, through a thirst for knowledge, learned much about me – how I think, respond and position philosophical considerations in life.
- As a gay man, I have learned the skills of standing up for rights, equality, fair treatment and inclusivity. In nursing this is what is often required for the benefit of our patients. The personal self and professional self in my view are explicitly interlinked. As a leader I want more than anything to be part of a system that provides the best learning experience to students; as a nurse I want nothing less than the same for our patients.

... AND FINALLY

We hope that you have found this book useful, and our own reflections are given as an encouragement to you and your careers. We are inspired as academics to be a part of the development of the future professional leaders in our nursing profession. We hope that is YOU!

Brian and Ruth

INDEX

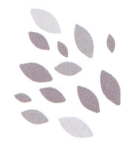

Note: Page numbers in **bold** indicate activities and page numbers in *italics* refer to figures and tables.